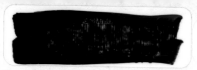

Sex Cells

The publisher gratefully acknowledges the generous support of the General Endowment Fund of the University of California Press Foundation.

Sex Cells

THE MEDICAL MARKET FOR EGGS AND SPERM

RENE ALMELING

UNIVERSITY OF CALIFORNIA PRESS
Berkeley   Los Angeles   London

University of California Press, one of the most distinguished university presses in the United States, enriches lives around the world by advancing scholarship in the humanities, social sciences, and natural sciences. Its activities are supported by the UC Press Foundation and by philanthropic contributions from individuals and institutions. For more information, visit www.ucpress.edu.

University of California Press
Berkeley and Los Angeles, California

University of California Press, Ltd.
London, England

Library of Congress Cataloging-in-Publication Data

Almeling, Rene
    Sex cells : the medical market for eggs and sperm / Rene Almeling.
        p. cm.
    Includes bibliographical references and index.
    ISBN 978-0-520-27095-4 (hardcover : alk. paper) —
    ISBN 978-0-520-27096-1 (pbk. : alk. paper)
    1. Artificial insemination, Human—Economic aspects. 2. Artificial insemination, Human—Moral and ethical aspects. 3. Infertility—Treatment—Economic aspects. 4. Surrogate motherhood—Economic aspects. I. Title.
    HQ761.A46 2011
    381'.45618178—dc22

                                                        2011008654

Manufactured in the United States of America

20 19 18 17 16 15 14 13 12 11
10 9 8 7 6 5 4 3 2 1

In keeping with a commitment to support environmentally responsible and sustainable printing practices, UC Press has printed this book on Rolland Enviro100, a 100% post-consumer fiber paper that is FSC certified, deinked, processed chlorine-free, and manufactured with renewable biogas energy. It is acid-free and EcoLogo certified.

Contents

Acknowledgments

As a nineteen-year-old undergraduate, I read an essay by Katha Pollitt on the Baby M surrogacy trial. I became fascinated by the complex issues associated with the prospect of women selling reproductive services and wrote a senior thesis under the wonderful mentorship of Elizabeth Long, the sociology professor who had assigned the essay. More than a decade later, this book is part of an ongoing attempt to sort through the questions raised by bodily commodification, and I am grateful for the chance to express my appreciation to all those who have made it possible.

First, a heartfelt thanks to the staff and donors at the programs where I conducted research. Each person I spoke with was so generous with their time, and I cannot thank them enough for their patience in answering my many questions.

I am also deeply grateful to my dissertation committee: Gail Klig-man, Ruth Milkman, Abigail Saguy, and Carole Browner. As chair of the committee, and from my first semester in graduate school, Gail has been an ideal mentor, spending time talking with me about ideas, providing detailed feedback on my writing, and inspiring me with her high stan-dards of scholarship. Early conversations with Ruth, Abigail, and Carole helped orient me to sociological and anthropological thinking on gen-der, work, medicine, and the body, and ever since, they have provided crucial intellectual guidance and enthusiasm for this project.

There are a number of scholars who have engaged with my research along the way, sharing useful insights and providing helpful comments. First and foremost in this category is Stefan Timmermans, who pro-vided detailed feedback on several of the chapters and was always avail-able to talk over snags in the writing process. I am fortunate to have met Kieran Healy while I was still working on my master's thesis (which eventually became Chapter 2), and ever since, he has been an absolutely essential interlocutor on this project. Both he and Diane Wolf read the entire book manuscript and provided excellent suggestions for refining it. Andrew Deener has provided extremely useful comments on more than one version of most chapters in this book. I thank Greta Krippner for conversations we had as I was crafting the dissertation proposal. Thanks also to the following people who provided helpful comments on various chapter drafts: Gabriel Abend, Jeffrey Alexander, Claudio Ben-zecry, Elizabeth Bernstein, Elizabeth Ettorre, John Evans, Adrian Favell, Carrie Friese, Kurtulus Gemici, Jerry Jacobs, Rob Jansen, Joanna Kempner, Kimberly Krawiec, Sandy Levitsky, Cameron MacDonald, Suzanne Pelka, Gabrielle Raley, Kevin Riley, Daisy Rooks, Barbara Katz Roth-man, Kristen Schilt, Beth Schneider, Sara Shostak, Elly Teman, Emily Wentzell, Owen Whooley, Viviana Zelizer, Lynne Zucker, and anony-mous reviewers for *American Sociological Review* and *New Genetics and Society*.

Research funding for this project came from the National Science Foundation, the UCLA Graduate Division, the UCLA Sociology Depart-ment, the UCLA Center for Society and Genetics, and the UCLA Center for the Study of Women. A postdoctoral fellowship from the Robert

Wood Johnson Foundation Scholars in Health Policy Research Program included time to revise the dissertation into a book, and while in residence at the UC Berkeley/UCSF site, I benefited from the mentorship of Dan Dohan, Charis Thompson, Joan Bloom, Carroll Estes, Neil Smelser, and John Ellwood. I completed the final draft of the book as a new faculty member in the sociology department at Yale, and I thank my colleagues for our conversations about the project. It has been a pleasure to work with Naomi Schneider at the University of California Press, which is home to many of the books on gender and reproduction that have shaped my thinking.

For their ability to manage any and all questions and problems, I am deeply appreciative of Marlies Dietrich and Linda Schulman (UCLA Sociology Department), Carlene Brown (UCLA Center for Society and Genetics), Seana Van Buren and Stacy Gallagher (Robert Wood Johnson Foundation's UC–Berkeley site), and Pam Colesworthy (Yale Sociology Department). Susan Paulukonis, Cecily Miller, Carmen Krol, Hae Jin Kang, Winifred Ko, and Christine Ilagan provided excellent research assistance. Lynda Klopatek efficiently and accurately transcribed the majority of the interviews.

Earlier versions of part of the Introduction and most of Chapter 2 were published as "Selling Genes, Selling Gender: Egg Agencies, Sperm Banks, and the Medical Market in Genetic Material" in the *American Sociological Review* 72 (2007): 319–340. A few paragraphs in Chapter 1 were included in "Gender and the Value of Bodily Goods: Commodification in Egg and Sperm Donation" in *Law and Contemporary Problems* 72 (2009): 37–58. An earlier version of Figure 2 in Chapter 2 was published in " 'Why do you want to be a donor?': Gender and the Production of Altruism in Egg and Sperm Donation" in *New Genetics and Society* 25 (2006): 143–157.

Thank you to the family and friends who hosted me as I traveled for research and writing: David Almeling, Warren and Veronika Ostergren, Briana Patterson and Chris Dente, Carla Eckhardt, and Matt Carrigan. Thanks also to all of those who e-mailed news stories and sent clippings over the years. My late grandmother, Lorraine Almeling, was particularly indefatigable in this regard, even writing to *The Oprah Winfrey Show* to request a transcript for an episode on sperm donation.

My parents, Guy Almeling and Linda Sebastian, probably never thought I would build on their professional interests in economics, health care, and psychology by writing a sociological study of the market for sex cells, but there is no question that their curiosity about the world has shaped me in more ways than I realize. I especially want to thank them for teaching me how to ask questions and how to listen to the answers.

For the last fifteen years, I have had the unbelievable good fortune of sharing my life with Jeff Ostergren. In a million different ways, he has been supportive of everything I ever wanted to do, and the words to properly acknowledge him do not exist.

Introduction

Rushing from class at the university to her job downtown, Megan tuned in to the radio and half listened to an advertisement calling on young women to give the gift of life. Her ears perked up on hearing that financial compensation would be offered to those who are caring, healthy, and willing to help infertile couples have a child. Thinking about the tuition bill that was coming due next semester, she decided to call for more information. The men at Megan's school hear a different kind of pitch. Flipping through the pages of the college newspaper, they might come across a cartoon drawing of sperm floating above a call for a few good men, those who are healthy, in their twenties or thirties, and in pursuit or possession of a university degree. The copy suggests that they put their sperm to work and "get paid for what you're already doing." These ads are for egg donors and sperm donors, women and men who are paid to provide sex cells to people who are using reproductive technologies to have children.

Unimaginable until the twentieth century, the practice of clinically transferring eggs and sperm from body to body is now part of a multibillion dollar market.[1] Hundreds of fertility clinics in the United States offer services ranging from artificial insemination to more complicated procedures such as *in vitro* fertilization (IVF), and they are dependent on a constant supply of sex cells for clients who do not have or cannot use their own eggs and sperm. Tens of thousands of children have been born as a result of such technologies, and the number of people attempting to conceive via assisted reproduction rises every year.[2]

Although it would be shocking to see a child listed for sale and it is illegal to sell one's organs, it is routine for egg and sperm donors to receive financial compensation. Payments to women in the United States range from a few thousand to tens of thousands of dollars, depending on the characteristics of the donor and the program where she is donating.[3] In contrast, there is much less variation in the rates paid to men; most sperm banks offer around $100 per sample.

Despite the monetary exchange, staffers in egg agencies and sperm banks consistently refer to this practice as "donation." Depending on the sex of the donor, though, there are subtle differences in how donation is understood, differences that are already apparent in the language of the ads mentioned above: egg donation is portrayed as an altruistic gift while sperm donation is considered an easy job. Given that eggs and sperm are similar kinds of cells—each contains half of the genetic material needed to create an embryo—what explains these different understandings?

The answer to this question is not reducible to biology or technology. In this book, I bring together sociological theories of the market with gendered theories of the body to create a framework for analyzing markets for bodily goods, both in terms of how such markets are organized and in how they are experienced. Eggs and sperm are parallel bodily goods. But they are produced by differently sexed bodies, and looking closely at this market reveals the extent to which it is shaped by economic and cultural understandings of biological sex differences as well as gendered expectations of women and men. The chapters that follow offer an inside look at egg agencies and sperm banks. Listening to the staff who organize the market and hearing from the donors who sustain it reveals the many ways in which the gendered framing of donation as a gift or a job matters: it influences how donation programs do business, and it profoundly affects the women and men whose sex cells are being purchased.

MARKETS FOR BODILY GOODS: FROM SEX TO CELLS

Commodification of the body—a process in which economic value is assigned to bodily services or goods—has long generated heated debates that only grow more intense as the number and kind of goods for sale increase. There is, of course, prostitution, the "oldest profession," which has undergone enormous changes in the last few decades as evolving transportation and communication technologies have provided new opportunities for people to buy and sell sex. In medicine, eighteenth-century scientists began to evince a ghoulish need for corpses to sustain and nurture their burgeoning knowledge of human anatomy. More recently, the development of surgical techniques and transplant medicine has fostered demand for various body parts, from blood and organs to bone marrow and even faces.[4] But it is in the realm of reproduction, where there has been an explosion in the use of medical technologies to have children, that some of the most pointed questions about markets for bodily goods have been raised.

Infertility, a condition barely spoken of at the beginning of the twentieth century, is now defined as a medical problem and routinely discussed on daytime talk shows and in the pages of the *New York Times*.[5] Affecting roughly 10% of the population, infertility can often be traced to physical problems such as blocked fallopian tubes or low sperm count. However, demographic trends and changing cultural norms have also contributed to an increased reliance on reproductive technologies. More women than ever are seeking higher education and participating in the labor force, and as a result, some choose to delay childbearing.[6] Gays and lesbians, whose reproductive decisions have become more visible as they advocate for rights associated with marriage and parenthood, are also increasingly turning to the medical profession for help in conceiving children.[7]

The technologies currently offered are the result of centuries of reproductive experimentation. The first attempts at artificial insemination began in the late 1700s, but it was more than a century before the use of *donated* sperm was reported in the medical literature. Today, insemination involves the use of a syringe to place semen into a woman's vagina or uterus. Vaginal inseminations are fairly simple, and some women opt to perform this procedure at home; however, intrauterine inseminations are typically performed in medical settings.[8]

Experiments with IVF began in the 1930s but did not result in a human birth until 1978, and success with *donated* eggs followed just a few years later.[9] Today, an IVF cycle involves a woman self-injecting fertility medications for several weeks, which stimulates the ovaries to produce multiple eggs that are then removed in outpatient surgery. Eggs and sperm (also called "gametes") are mixed together in the lab, and if viable embryos result, a few are placed in the woman's uterus.[10] People who use insemination or IVF to conceive generally prefer to use their own eggs or sperm, but some must turn to egg and/or sperm donors. Those who cannot sustain a pregnancy might opt to engage the gestational services of a surrogate mother.[11]

In undergoing the first part of an IVF cycle, egg donors face short-term risks associated with both the fertility drugs and the egg retrieval surgery, risks that include ovarian hyperstimulation syndrome, infection, bleeding, and complications from the anesthesia. The American Society for Reproductive Medicine (ASRM) estimates the risk of serious complications to be around 1%, and the few empirical studies that have been conducted find similar rates.[12] There is very little research on the long-term effects of undergoing IVF, which has led to calls for an egg donor registry to track young women who are exposed to fertility medications early in life.[13]

There are no physical risks associated with sperm donation, but men's activities are restricted for a much longer period of time than egg donors'. Most programs require that men commit to producing samples by masturbating at the sperm bank at least once a week for an entire year, and each donation must be preceded by two days of abstinence from sexual activity. If the sample meets bank standards for sperm count and semen volume, it will be frozen and stored in the bank's offices until it is purchased by recipients for use in insemination.

The United States has responded to technological interventions in reproduction with far less regulation than other countries. For example, Britain's Warnock Report, issued in 1984, resulted in the Human Fertilization and Embryology Authority (HFEA), which monitors and makes policy on all aspects of assisted reproduction.[14] The HFEA sets compensation for egg and sperm donors at very low levels, and in 2005, it eliminated anonymous donation, requiring that identifying information about donors be shared with offspring at age eighteen. In contrast, the United States' laissez-faire approach has permitted the existence of fairly open markets for reproductive goods and services. Starting in 1992, Congress required that fertility clinics report the number of procedures performed each year as well as what proportion are successful. But there are no federal requirements regarding payments to donors, and ethical determinations about other aspects of egg and sperm donation are left to professional societies such as ASRM, which have very little power to enforce the guidelines they issue.[15]

THEORIZING BODILY COMMODIFICATION

The issue of bodily commodification has drawn sustained attention from scholars in many disciplines, from law, philosophy, and ethics to history, sociology, and anthropology. Despite all this attention, though, there remains a schism in the wide-ranging literature. On one side, scholars conceptualize commodification as uniform; the simple fact that money is exchanged for all or part of a human being is fundamental in shaping the market. On the other side, scholars contend that the exchange of money for bodily goods and services is a variable social process; it can proceed in many different ways and be imbued with many different meanings.

The first view has a longer history and more adherents. There are a few in this camp who are unabashedly pro-commodification, arguing for open markets for sex, children, organs, and the like.[16] But the vast majority of scholars in this area have been sharply critical of assigning economic value to bodies, contending that the effects of doing so are uniformly negative. Richard Titmuss' classic study of blood donation provides just one example. When he was conducting research in the 1960s, the United States relied on a hodgepodge system of paid and voluntary donors, which he compared with the wholly voluntary, centralized blood collection system in the United Kingdom. Titmuss concluded that altruism-based systems like the UK's produce safer blood and are morally preferable to payment-based systems, writing, "blood as a living tissue may now constitute in Western societies one of the ultimate tests of where the 'social' begins and the 'economic' ends."[17]

Writing about egg donation twenty-five years later, bioethicist Thomas Murray revealed a similarly dichotomous view of society and economy when he asks,

> Are children more likely to flourish in a culture where making children is governed by the same rules that govern the making of automobiles or VCRs? Or is their flourishing more assured in a culture where making children . . . is treated as a sphere separate from the marketplace? A sphere governed by the ethics of gift and relationship, not contract and commerce?[18]

Indeed, deeply embedded in this first view is the assumption that bodily commodification is harmful, both for the society and for the individual. In tracing the stigma associated with earning money through the use of one's body from the ancient Greeks to the present, philosopher Martha Nussbaum bluntly summarizes the prevailing opinion. "It is widely believed . . . that taking money or entering into contracts in connection with the use of one's sexual and reproductive capacities is genuinely bad."[19] In the following laundry list, Titmuss specified all the ways in which he believes paying for blood produces negative effects.

> The commercialization of blood and donor relationships represses the expression of altruism, erodes the sense of community, lowers scientific standards, limits both personal and professional freedoms, sanctions the

making of profits in hospitals and clinical laboratories, legalizes hostility between doctor and patient, subjects critical areas of medicine to the laws of the marketplace, places immense social costs on those least able to bear them—the poor, the sick, and the inept—increases the danger of unethical behavior in various sectors of medical science and practice, and results in situations in which proportionately more and more blood is supplied by the poor, the unskilled, the unemployed. . . ."[20]

In sum, abstract distinctions—economic/social and commodity/gift— undergird this first view of commodification as uniformly degrading: when the market expands to incorporate bodily goods, social relations are invariably threatened.

On the other side of the schism in this literature is a view based on the opposite assumption, which is that markets and social life are inextricably intertwined. Economic processes are shaped by social factors and vice versa. One leading proponent of this second view is Viviana Zelizer, a sociologist whose research has spanned the emerging market for life insurance, the changing cultural and economic value of children, and the social and legal interpretations of monetary exchanges in intimate relationships.[21] Based on this research, she has formulated a sociological model of markets in which economic, cultural, and structural factors interact. Zelizer notes, "As an interactive model, it precludes not only economic absolutism but also cultural determinism or social structural reductionism in the analysis of economic processes."[22]

In allowing for the possibility of variation in how markets are configured, this model opens up the theoretical prospect that commodification can have various and multiple effects on those who participate in such markets. In this way, the work of Zelizer and others contests the idea that commodification is inherently or solely detrimental. For example, legal scholar Margaret Jane Radin has endeavored to better understand the "complexities of commodification as we experience it. These complexities include the plurality of meanings of any particular interaction, the dynamic nature of these meanings (their instability), and the possible effects (good or ill) in the world of either promoting or trying to forestall a commodified understanding of something that we have previously valued in a noneconomic way."[23] Likewise, Kieran Healy's sociological analyses of blood and organ donation challenge normative assumptions, such as those in Titmuss' work, about the evils of the marketplace and the benefits of gift exchange. Healy concludes, "The idea that markets inevitably corrupt is not tenable precisely *because* they are embedded within social relations, cultural categories, and institutional routines."[24]

Debates about commodification are so extensive because they are so crucial, and thus it is important to directly address this schism. *Is the process of bodily commodification uniform or variable? If there is variation in how markets for bodily goods are organized, to what extent does that variation affect the experience of being paid for bodily goods?* Asking the question in this way builds upon previous research but is innovative in that it clearly delineates two aspects of bodily commodification: the *organization* of the market and the *experience* of the market. Scholars who assume commodification is uniform have not had cause to ask these questions, while those who attend to variation have generally focused on the organization of markets, paying less attention to the embodied experience of commodification. In the next two sections, I develop a theoretical framework to address each of these two levels of analysis.

ORGANIZING THE MARKET: SEX, GENDER, AND THE VALUE OF BODILY GOODS

In bringing together economic, cultural, and structural factors, Zelizer's sociological model of a market is a useful starting point, but to analyze the organization of markets for bodily goods, I find it necessary to incorporate biological factors into the framework. Doing so allows for the explicit accounting of different kinds of bodies and different kinds of bodily goods in studies of bodily commodification. In this book, I focus on a particular kind of bodily difference, that of sex. So, in this case, taking biological factors into consideration involves conceptualizing eggs and sperm as cells that are associated with female and male bodies, as well as gendered expectations of women and men.

Here, I am drawing on a long-standing distinction in feminist theory between "sex," which is defined as biological differences between females and males, and "gender," which is defined as the cultural meanings attributed to those biological differences.[25] In general, social scientists have paid more attention to gender and downplayed biological sex differences. However, as Sylvia Yanagisako and Jane Collier note, the failure to analyze sex is a mistake because "having conceded sex differences to biology in the interest of establishing our scholarly authority over socially and culturally constituted gender differences, we have limited our project and legitimized assumptions about sexual difference that return to haunt our theories of gender."[26]

The challenge lies in incorporating biological factors into sociological analyses without reverting to an essentialist tautology, in which sex differences are the beginning and end of explanations for gender inequality. As a way out of this conundrum, Judith Butler suggests a social constructionist approach that acknowledges bodily differences but contends that bodies are anything but empty, "natural" vessels waiting to be filled with cultural meaning. Instead, she argues that bodies themselves (their differences and similarities) cannot be understood outside of social processes, which means that sex differences are just as socially constructed as gender differences.[27] This perspective, with its analytical openness to variation in how sex is constructed—or more specifically for the purposes of this study, in how biology is valued—sits well within a theoretical framework that allows for variation in how biological factors come together with cultural factors, structural factors, and economic factors to shape markets.

If the valuation of biology is inseparable from these other factors, then bodies do not contain inherent and unchanging value, and it becomes important to think through the various ways in which the worth of sex cells might be established. The first possibility is that eggs and sperm will be equally valued. This may be due to *biological* symmetry, in that eggs and sperm each contain twenty-three chromosomes and creating an embryo requires one egg from one woman and one sperm from one man. Or it may result from *structural* symmetry, in that both egg and sperm donors are recruited by donation programs to produce genetic material for sale to recipient clients, who will conceive children to whom the donors have no responsibility.

The second possibility is that eggs and sperm will be differently valued. After all, these cells are produced by differently sexed bodies. Female bodies have a limited supply of eggs while men's supply of sperm is continually replenished, and extracting eggs entails risk and pain that extracting sperm does not. These *biological* differences may result in an understanding of eggs as a scarce resource, and *economic* mechanisms associated with the pressures of supply and demand may result in women's donation being more highly valued than men's.

Shifting the emphasis to *cultural* and *structural* factors suggests the opposite outcome: broader patterns of gender inequality will result in men's donation being more highly valued than women's. In her research on descriptions of eggs and sperm in medical textbooks, Emily Martin finds that "cultural ideas about passive females and heroic males [are imported] into the 'personalities' of gametes."[28] If a similar pattern holds in the market for sex cells, sperm will be more valued than eggs. Another possibility is that egg agencies and sperm banks consider donors to be reproductive service workers. Given that there is persistent income inequality by sex, trends that are exacerbated in service work and care work,[29] it is possible that sperm donors will be more valued than egg donors.

However, it may be *cultural* norms associated with the family, not the workplace, that influence processes of valuation in this market, as these bodily goods are intended to help people have children. Traditionally, ideals of femininity and motherhood have portrayed women as denizens of the private sphere who are selfless, caring, and devoted to others, while ideals of masculinity and fatherhood situate men as hardworking, emotionally distant breadwinners who inhabit the public sphere. These distinctions are nicely summed up by Julie Nelson and Paula England, who write that "women, love, altruism and the family are, as a group, [viewed as] radically separate and opposite from men, self-interested rationality, work and market exchange."[30] Thus, it is possible that women donating eggs will be perceived as altruistic helpers who want nothing more than for recipients to have families, while men donating sperm will be construed as employees performing a job with little care for the bank's customers.

In the first part of the book, I demonstrate how these factors—biological bodies, economic mechanisms, and gendered cultural norms—interact within the structural context of donation programs to produce variation in the organization of the market, both in terms of how sex cells are valued and in the expectations placed on egg and sperm donors. The end result is that eggs are more highly valued than sperm, and egg donation is understood as a gift while sperm donation is considered a job. The next question is whether such variation influences women's and men's experiences of bodily commodification.

EXPERIENCING THE MARKET: GIFT RHETORIC, EMOTIONAL LABOR, AND BEING A PAID DONOR

The market for sex cells incorporates both financial compensation and the language of donation, a combination that appears oxymoronic at first glance. The reason that paid donation sounds so incongruous is the longstanding assumption that gifts and commodities are not only completely distinct from one another, but are also very different kinds of things. Arjun Appadurai traced this assumption among social scientists to the different legacies of Marcel Mauss and Karl Marx, providing the following summary.

> Gifts, and the spirit of reciprocity, sociability, and spontaneity in which they are typically exchanged, usually are starkly opposed to the profit-oriented, self-centered, and calculated spirit that fires the circulation of commodities. Further, where gifts link things to persons and embed the flow of things in the flow of social relations, commodities are held to represent the drive—largely free of moral or cultural constraints—of goods for one another, a drive mediated by money and not by sociality.[31]

In an echo of Zelizer's argument, Appadurai considers this dichotomy to be an oversimplified depiction of economic life, and he has encouraged scholars to trace the social life of things. In particular, he underscores the possibility that the same thing can sometimes be both a gift and a commodity, albeit at different points in its trajectory. Lesley Sharp pushes this point further, drawing on research in organ donation to contend that multiple understandings of the same bodily good might be operating at the *same* time, especially in medical settings. For the deceased's kin, a donated organ is a part of the family that lives on; for the recipient, it is a lifesaving gift; for the doctors, it is a valuable commodity that should not be "wasted" on an undeserving recipient. Sharp concludes, "The language of gift exchange may obscure capitalist forms of commodification. In other words, two models of commodification might be at work simultaneously, one more akin to Mauss's understanding of the symbolically charged gift and reciprocity, the other to Marx's notion of commodities as goods produced under the alienating conditions of capitalism."[32]

The question is whether these various understandings *matter* for the people whose bodies are being commodified. What happens when paid donation is considered to be more of a gift or more of a job? Shifting the focus from determining which things are actually gifts or actually commodities to comparing the use of gift rhetoric and commodity rhetoric makes possible an analysis of whether commodified exchange can be experienced in different ways.[33]

The first possibility is that framing donation as a gift or a job makes no difference whatsoever. It is merely language that "obscures," to use Sharp's word, what is really going on. This is a common theoretical vision of bodily commodification, one that also appears in Nancy Scheper-Hughes' definition of it as "encompassing all capitalized economic relations between humans in which human bodies are the token of economic exchanges that are often *masked* by something else – love, altruism, pleasure, kindness."[34] These scholars echo the view of Titmuss and others that the monetary exchange is fundamental, that commodification is inherently objectifying and alienating, and calling it something else does nothing to change the experience of being paid for bodily goods.

The second possibility is that these gendered frames do have consequences. Given that gift exchange is traditionally associated with affective ties and reciprocity while commodified exchange is marked by contractual relations that conclude when payment is rendered, it is possible that even just the use of gift language evokes a sense of sociability, a sense of connection between donor and recipient that is more durable and lasting than would be expected given the monetary exchange. This is especially plausible in a market for genetic material, as eggs and sperm

are purchased in the hopes of conceiving children. Our culture's emphasis on biogenetic ties in defining kinship may mean that donors are considered more as family than as strangers.

However, forging such connections may result in the expectation that
donors and recipients demonstrate care and concern for one another, a
form of emotional work. Arlie Hochschild originally formulated the concept of "emotional labor" in her study comparing female flight attendants,
who had to exhibit empathy for the customer's every concern, with male
debt collectors, who had to manufacture anger with debtors over the
phone. Subsequent studies have revealed that these sorts of gendered
expectations for emotional work appear in many kinds of employment,
and they are based in large part on the cultural norms of nurturing
femininity and distant masculinity discussed in the previous section.[35]

More recent research on emotional labor suggests that it may be experienced as more than just coercive and alienating. In a study of nursing
home workers, Steven Lopez finds that meaningful interactions can result from "organizational attempts to create hospitable conditions for the
development of caring relationships between service providers and recipients."[36] This raises the possibility that instilling an emotional connection between gamete donor and recipient may forestall feelings of
alienation, in that both parties are offered an alternative narrative to the
stigmatized story of handing over cash for body parts.

Since the dominant assumption has been that bodily commodification
is inherently and uniformly degrading, there has been relatively little
empirical research on the experiences of those who participate in such
markets, including the market for sex cells.[37] There is a rich tradition of
sociological and anthropological research on reproduction, some of which
includes discussions of commodification, but most of it centers on pregnancy, abortion, and birth, so there is little known about men's experiences in this realm.[38] In general, there has been less concern about the
commodification of men's bodies.[39]

Thus, I devote the second part of the book to analyzing how egg
and sperm donors experience bodily commodification. First, I examine
how they describe the physical aspects of donation, assessing whether
being paid to undergo IVF or engage in routine masturbation alters the

experience of these embodied processes. Second, I compare how egg and sperm donors define the money they receive with special attention to whether they consider it a gift for the gift they have given or wages for a job well done. Third, I look at how women and men respond to the possibility that biological offspring may result from their donations and analyze whether they identify their genetic connection as familial. Through close empirical attention to what happens when commodified exchange is mixed with gift rhetoric and when it is not, I find that the simple fact of payment does not solely determine the experience of commodification. Instead, I argue that organizing paid donation as a gift or a job has real consequences; it affects egg and sperm donors' physical experiences, as well as how they conceptualize what it is they are being paid to do.

DATA AND METHODS

To study how the medical market for sex cells is organized and experienced, I collected data on egg and sperm donation in the United States. Most of the data come from six donation programs, where I interviewed a total of forty-five staff members, nineteen egg donors, and twenty sperm donors between 2002 and 2006. These six programs vary in terms of which gametes they provide (eggs or sperm or both), tax status, size, geographic location, and longevity (see Table 1).

CryoCorp is one of the oldest and largest commercial sperm banks. It was started by a physician in the 1970s to serve infertile couples. OvaCorp is one of the oldest and largest commercial egg agencies. It expanded on a successful surrogacy business in the late 1980s to offer egg donation. Both programs run several offices in different parts of the country, but my research was limited to their West Coast locations. (All programs and people have been assigned pseudonyms. CryoCorp and OvaCorp have similar names not because of any relationship between the two programs but to indicate the symmetry in their organizational characteristics and their status as industry leaders.)

Western Sperm Bank is the only nonprofit sperm bank in the United States. With roots in the feminist women's health movement, it opened

Table 1 Overview of Donation Program Characteristics and Data Collection

	CryoCorp	Western Sperm Bank	OvaCorp	Creative Beginnings	Gametes Inc.	University Fertility Services
Program characteristics						
Gametes offered	Sperm	Sperm	Eggs	Eggs	Sperm, Eggs	Sperm, Eggs
Type	Commercial	Nonprofit	Commercial	Commercial	Commercial	University
Size	Large	Small	Large	Medium	Large	Small
Location	West	West	West	West	Southeast	Southeast
Founded	1977	1982	1989	1999	1975 (Sperm) 2003 (Eggs)	1985 (Sperm) 1993 (Eggs)
Data collected						
Years	2002, 2006	2002, 2004	2002	2002	2006	2005, 2006
Interviews	10 Staff	4 Staff 6 Sperm Donors	5 Staff 5 Egg Donors	7 Staff 6 Egg Donors	11 Staff 6 Egg Donors 14 Sperm Donors	8 Staff 2 Egg Donors
Observation			1 Day	6 Days	7 Days	7 Days
Donor profiles	125 Sperm	44 Sperm	466 Egg	129 Egg	112 Sperm 75 Egg	57 Sperm 149 Egg

in the early 1980s and maintains a small program on the West Coast. Creative Beginnings is a commercial egg agency on the West Coast that had been open for just a few years, but the founder/executive director had worked in infertility clinics for several decades. Gametes Inc., located in the Southeast, opened in the 1970s as a sperm bank and is similar to CryoCorp in age and size. However, it differs from CryoCorp in that it offers both sperm and eggs; it expanded on its established sperm bank business by opening an egg agency in the early 2000s. University Fertility Services is also located in the Southeast, and it is part of a major research university's department of obstetrics and gynecology. In an off-site women's health clinic designed for those with private insurance, the physicians and nurses run a small sperm and egg donation program to serve their infertility patients.[40]

In each of these six programs, I interviewed staff at all levels, including those with decision-making authority, such as founders and executive directors, and those who have the most contact with donors, including coordinators, office assistants, and lab technicians.[41] I asked open-ended questions about donor recruitment, the procedures for screening and monitoring those who were accepted into the program, payment protocols, and how the staff would define a "good donor" as well as reasons why applicants might be rejected. Most of the interviews with staff lasted between thirty and sixty minutes, but a few were as short as fifteen minutes, and some went on for several hours over several meetings.

My request to interview donors in these same programs was granted in all four egg agencies, but I was only able to interview sperm donors from two of the four sperm banks.[42] At Creative Beginnings and University Fertility Services' egg donation program, I selected donors to interview. At Gametes Inc., the staff asked all of the sperm donors who came by the week I was there whether they would be willing to speak with me. At OvaCorp, Western Sperm Bank, and Gametes Inc.'s egg donation program, the donor coordinator chose a group of donors for me to contact after checking in with them first about their willingness to be interviewed. To the extent possible, I asked the donor coordinators to select donors of different ages, racial/ethnic backgrounds, occupations, and parental status (i.e., whether the donor had children of his/her own).

In total, I spoke with nineteen egg donors and twenty sperm donors, ranging in age from 19 to 46. Many donors were still in school, and both those who were students and those who were not had a wide variety of occupations. The majority of donors were single. Seven women and two men had children of their own (see Appendix A for more information about the donors' characteristics). Nearly all of the sperm donors are "identity release," meaning they have agreed to let the sperm bank share identifying information with interested offspring after the children turn eighteen.[43] (Egg donation programs do not generally offer identity-release programs.)

As I was interested in whether the experience of donation changed over time, I interviewed donors who were at various stages in the process: those who had applied to donate but not yet started, those who were in the midst of donating, and those who had donated several years before our interview. I asked open-ended questions about their experiences, including how they first decided to pursue donation, what they thought of the screening process, where donation fit into their daily lives and their financial situations, and about their relationships with program staff, recipients, and offspring. The average egg donor interview lasted a little more than ninety minutes while the average sperm donor interview lasted about sixty minutes.[44]

From the files and websites of these same six programs, I collected more than a thousand donor profiles, which are designed to help recipients choose a donor but which also provide a demographic portrait of each program (see Appendix B). In programs that allowed it, I also spent several days observing daily business practices with a focus on how staff interacted with one another, with donors, and with recipients. The observations allowed me to compare what the staff reported in interviews with how they responded to everyday situations. I usually had my tape recorder running, and I jotted brief notes that I wrote up as more extensive field notes at the end of each day. I also gathered written materials such as office protocols, advertisements for donors, legal contracts, and informed consent forms.

In addition to research at contemporary donation programs, I studied the historical development of the market for sex cells. Beginning in 2005,

I conducted historical interviews with prominent physician–researchers and others who had been in the field of assisted reproduction for decades. Many worked in Southern California, a hotbed of both technological developments in assisted reproduction and their commercialization. Those who are mentioned in this book include a university-based physician–researcher who has served as president of ASRM and editor of *Fertility and Sterility*; a second physician–researcher who pioneered IVF with egg donation at a university before starting his own fertility practice and later served as president of the Society for Assisted Reproductive Technology (SART) (the nurse-coordinator who ran this physician's egg donation program in the late 1980s opened Creative Beginnings in the late 1990s); a third physician–researcher who has published widely about egg donation since the mid-1980s and who is currently chief of reproductive endocrinology and infertility at his university; and a therapist who founded a commercial egg agency that was one of the earliest and is now among the largest programs in the country. Most of these interviews lasted between thirty and sixty minutes.

To supplement these historical interviews, I read articles published in *Fertility and Sterility,* starting with its inception in 1950 and going through 2005, both to verify dates and also to gather information about how donation happened in other times and places. I searched LexisNexis for newspaper and magazine articles about the six donation programs where I did research. I also attended several medical conferences to observe clinicians discussing gamete donation. Finally, to analyze the visual and linguistic strategies used to recruit egg and sperm donors, I collected a national sample of newspaper advertisements from top universities and major media markets in 2006.

All of the interviews were conducted in person, recorded, transcribed in full, and entered into Nvivo, a software program that facilitates coding. To code the staff interviews, I relied on a chronological accounting of the donation process, which is most clearly visible in the structure of Chapter 2. For the donor interviews, I created forty codes based on my theoretical interests and themes that emerged from reading the transcripts.[45] I analyzed the interviews, observations, and historical materials with several different themes in mind, including the relationship between the historical development of the market and its contemporary organization, the organization of the donation process in different kinds of programs, and how different kinds of donors experienced bodily commodification. Most of the interview excerpts from staff, donors, and founders have been edited for brevity and clarity.

OVERVIEW OF THE BOOK

The first part of the book examines the organization of the market for sex cells, and the second part of the book analyzes egg and sperm donors' experiences in that market. Chapter 1 traces the emergence of the market for sperm and eggs, from the secretive history of artificial insemination at the beginning of the twentieth century to the development of IVF with donated eggs in the 1980s. Nested within this broader history, I explore the development of organizational protocols for managing the production of bodily goods in each of the six donation programs where I did research. Physicians running the earliest sperm banks emphasized anonymity and considered donation a quick task to be performed in exchange for cash. This provided an already-established model of gamete donation by the time it became possible for women to provide eggs, but physicians had different expectations for egg donors than they had had for sperm donors. They relaxed their requirements for anonymity and sought altruistic women who were donating for the "right reasons," that is, women who wanted to help infertile couples have families.

As physicians ceded control over the procurement of sex cells to commercial agencies, these gendered understandings of donation carried over into contemporary programs. Chapter 2 is a detailed comparison of two sperm banks and two egg agencies, where staff rely on extensive screening rubrics in determining who is allowed to be a donor and assign economic value to cells based on the type of person producing them. Drawing on cultural ideals of maternal femininity and paternal masculinity, staff frame egg donation as a gift and sperm donation as a job. This rhetoric combines with systematically different strategies for managing the monetary exchange to produce gender-specific regimes of bodily commodification.

Turning to the donors, Chapter 3 describes how they incorporate donation into their daily lives: women managing their bodies through the
shots and surgery of IVF and men managing their bodies through routine
masturbation and abstinence. In conversation with previous research, I
look at how infertile women and egg donors talk about IVF and find that
the embodied experience of this technology differs if women are doing it
for pregnancy or for profit. Analogously, I analyze how men experience
masturbation if they are doing so for pleasure or for profit and find that
being a sperm donor requires a surprising amount of bodily discipline.

Turning from the donors' physical experiences to how they conceptualize the money they receive, Chapter 4 reveals that most women and
men are motivated to donate by the prospect of financial compensation,
and they spend the money in similar ways. However, as they go through
the process of donation and interact with staff, egg donors mobilize gift
rhetoric in defining what it is they are being paid to do while sperm donors rely on employment rhetoric in categorizing donation as a job. More
than just language that "obscures" or "masks" what is really going on,
these gendered conceptualizations of donation have consequences.
Women talk with pride about the "huge" gift they are giving to recipients, and men reference feelings of alienation in defining themselves as
"assets" or "resources" for the sperm bank.

In Chapter 5, I explore the extent to which donors feel connected to the
children who result from their donations. Despite their equivalent genetic
contribution to offspring, sperm donors think of themselves as fathers to
these children while egg donors are adamant that they are not mothers.
Egg donors define their contribution as "just an egg," a fragmented understanding of reproduction that is buttressed by the connection they feel
with recipients, whom they identify as the mothers. Sperm donors hear
little about recipients and are encouraged to sign up for identity-release
programs, which underscore the importance of men's genetic contribution.
In seeing themselves as integral to the lives of offspring, sperm donors reflect broader Western notions of the male role in reproduction as primary.

Eggs and sperm are similar kinds of bodily goods, but they are produced by differently sexed bodies, and this results in different donation
processes and different associations with cultural norms of gender. It is

this combination of similarity and difference that makes possible a systematic study of variation in how bodily commodification is organized and experienced. In medicalized donation programs, cultural and economic understandings of the reproductive body combine to produce a market in which women are paid thousands of dollars to give the gift of life while men are paid piece rate based on bodily performance. In the Conclusion, I return to the themes introduced here to offer an explanation for why it is that egg donation is considered a gift and sperm donation a job, contending that it is not just sex cells on offer but visions of traditional American femininity and masculinity, and more precisely, motherhood and fatherhood. Building on the findings from this study, I propose a new way of theorizing bodily commodification, which raises new questions that can best be answered with detailed, empirical studies of what exactly happens when people are paid for parts of their bodies.

PART ONE Organizing the Market

ONE Characterizing the Material

In 1909, a short article appeared in *Medical World*, a "practical medical monthly." The author, Addison Hard, described a scene from twenty-five years before, when he and fellow medical students were observing Dr. William Pancoast's practice in Philadelphia. The doctor was approached by a wealthy merchant and his wife who confided their difficulties in conceiving a child. After discovering that the merchant had no sperm in his semen, one of the students joked that it was time to "call in the hired man." The doctor requested a sperm sample from the "best-looking member of the class" but did not inform the couple of his plans. He called the merchant's wife into his office, administered chloroform, and inseminated her with the student's sperm sample. She gave birth to a healthy baby boy. Eventually, Dr. Pancoast informed the merchant, who was "delighted with the idea," but both decided not to tell his wife.[1]

Several aspects of this story foreshadow the organization of gamete donation in the United States, including the centrality and power of physicians, the endemic secrecy associated with what was considered a morally questionable practice, and the selection of donors thought to have superior qualities. In tracing the development of the medical market for sex cells, from its earliest incarnations to the present day, focusing on *information*—what physicians wanted to know about the men and women providing gametes as well as what they shared with recipients— reveals stark differences in the management of sperm and egg donation. In this chapter, I look at how the process of characterizing reproductive material and the people donating that material have changed over time.

SPERM: FROM MEDICAL SERVICE TO COMMERCIAL PRODUCT

As the nineteenth century gave way to the twentieth, physicians began coupling the technology of artificial insemination with the use of donated sperm, but they did not trumpet the availability of this service, either to patients or to other physicians. An American doctor writing in the 1930s reported finding just a few scattered articles about this "therapy" for male infertility in the medical literature.[2] In part, this was due to continuing questions about its legality, as there had been court rulings defining the use of donated sperm as adulterous and the offspring as illegitimate. The rulings concerned physicians in the newly formed American Society for the Study of Sterility (later the American Fertility Society and now the American Society for Reproductive Medicine), who singled out artificial insemination as one of the issues they intended to address in the very first issue of their journal, *Fertility and Sterility*, published in 1950.[3]

In fact, the nascent society had already formed a special committee headed by Alan Guttmacher, who had also been an advocate for access to birth control and abortion. A survey of the society's ninety-six members in 1947 revealed that the majority approved of donor insemination, and the forty-four physicians who reported offering it had inseminated a total of 568 women that year.[4] Just a few years later, the following resolution was overwhelmingly approved by the full membership.

> If it is in harmony with the beliefs of the couple and the doctor, donor artificial insemination is a completely ethical, moral, and desirable form of medical therapy. Conditions under which donor artificial insemination is acceptable include:
>
> 1. Urgent desire of the couple to have such therapy applied to the solution of their infertility problem.
> 2. Careful selection by the physician of a biologically and genetically satisfactory donor.[5]
> 3. The opinion of the physician, after thorough study, that the couple will make desirable parents.[6]

Publicized as one of the society's first major policy statements, it was covered by the *New York Times, Reader's Digest,* and *McCall's.*[7]

In defining sperm donation as a medical therapy, physicians sought to dismiss the claims of legal and moral authorities over the procedure in a process that Peter Conrad has labeled "medicalization." Such appeals to the professional and cultural power of medicine were particularly effective in the middle of the twentieth century, a period known as the "golden age" of medicine, when physicians retained wide latitude in defining matters of health and the body, including reproduction.[8]

To find "biologically and genetically satisfactory" donors, physicians generally looked to the ranks of medical students and residents, calling them in as necessary to provide a fresh sample in exchange for a small fee.[9] For each sample, donors were paid around $20 to $35, a rate that did not change much over the course of the twentieth century.[10] In matching donors with recipients, the 1947 survey demonstrated that physicians prioritized "physical resemblance" to the recipient's husband, with "racial identity" at the top of the list while many also attempted "mental similarity" and "religious equality."[11] Physicians undertook these efforts to facilitate the recipient couples' ability to keep donor insemination a secret, and physical resemblance to the husband remained paramount over the years. Additional criteria for the donor eventually came to include minimum sperm count, satisfactory family health history, and tests for sexually transmitted diseases.[12]

Doctors maintained strict anonymity between donors and recipients, leading some support staff, often women working as nurses or secretaries, to conduct surreptitious screening of the men who applied to donate. CryoCorp, now one of the largest sperm banks in the country, was founded by a physician in the 1970s, and here he explains his initial procedures for screening donors.

Founder: We would advertise at [the university], and then I would do a physical on a donor, a history. I would get a sperm count, freeze the sample to see if it was good when we recovered it.

Rene: What kind of things were you looking for in that screening?
Founder: Evidence of congenital anomalies, sexually transmitted diseases, some reason they should not be a donor. Medications, drugs, sometimes arrogance, ugly, father with diabetes or heart attack, sibling that died unexpectedly.

Rene: If they were ugly or arrogant?
Founder: With me, I was working up a donor who seemed acceptable. He was a college student, had a good semen analysis. But when he left my office, the three women working for me at the time put their head in and said, "Doctor, you can accept him, but we're never going to send his sperm out. He's ugly." Okay, something I didn't put on my criteria at the time, but I had three somewhat articulate, vocal, outspoken women that let me know what they thought. They did not want ugly donors. I guess in some way they could identify, "If I don't want him, I'm not going to have him in here." So they reached the point that they would actually screen the donors to make sure that they weren't ugly or something just unappealing about them. Not that unappealing is a genetic trait.

In another donation program across the country, a laboratory technician described a similar dynamic. "Anybody that was butt-ugly, there was something wrong with his semen analysis [laughs]. We tried to keep them average- to good-looking. I just feel like the patients thought that was real important." In response to my question about whether she spoke to the physician about it, she explained, "This was kind of happening between the nurse and me. Generally we pretty much agreed to give a bad post-thaw motility. If I just let [the sperm sample] sit for a couple hours instead of checking it within five minutes, it'd make a big difference."

It was not until the last quarter of the twentieth century that physicians began to cede control of donor selection to commercial sperm banks like CryoCorp. Doctors had long been suspicious of such banks, raising questions about the commercialization of sperm donation that are similar in tone to Titmuss' warnings about blood donation.[13] For example, here is part of a commentary by Guttmacher in a 1958 issue of *Fertility and Sterility*.

> I must raise my voice against semen banks . . . The chronic, professional blood donor is hardly the Platonic image of an ideal source of the male element in the process of fertilization. A physician must choose the donor with the specific requirements of each insemination in sharp focus and not on a mass basis . . . I doubt that a semen bank with its assembly-line mechanisms could and would do the assignment satisfactorily. Experience has shown me that the most trustworthy donors are married house-staff physicians or medical students who have already fathered normal children. They are most likely to disbar themselves as donors for eugenic or health reasons. It is unnecessary to emphasize to readers of this Journal that in the ethical sense, whenever a physician performs donor insemination he is substituting for the Creator. This is no mean responsibility.[14]

Relying on the rhetoric of industry ("mass basis" and "assembly-line mechanisms"), Guttmacher underscores the importance of physician control in ensuring quality providers of the "male element."

The first commercial banks did not open until the 1970s, offering frozen sperm stored in tanks of liquid nitrogen, but they struggled against the perception that frozen-and-thawed sperm resulted in lower rates of conception than "fresh" sperm.[15] As a result, most physicians continued to use fresh sperm from donors they selected themselves, which distinguished them from clinicians in other countries. For example, France had more frozen sperm banks than the much larger United States, because

American doctors preferred to control all aspects of donor insemination, despite the scheduling inconveniences associated with using fresh samples.[16]

The advent of the AIDS epidemic changed this calculus, however, in that frozen sperm could be quarantined, making it possible to wait for several months after a donation before testing the donor again for HIV. But even as the threat of AIDS became more clear in the 1980s, physicians were loath to give up control. In a 1986 article introducing the American Fertility Society's latest guidelines regarding donor insemination, the past president of the society bucks the recommendations of the American Association of Tissue Banks, concluding that patients would be best served by the continued use of fresh semen provided by physician-screened donors. He specifically references distrust of commercial banks, the greater chance of pregnancy with fresh sperm, and the importance of physician control.[17]

Given the strong and continuing endorsement of fresh sperm by the major professional association in the field, it is not surprising that a 1987 survey of physicians found 22% continued to rely solely upon fresh semen for donor insemination.[18] It was not until 1988 that the Centers for Disease Control and Prevention (CDC) and the Food and Drug Administration (FDA) recommended, but still did not require, the use of frozen sperm, and then the American Fertility Society updated its 1986 guidelines, stating "the use of fresh semen is no longer warranted." Between 1986 and 1989, six women in the United States were infected with HIV after being inseminated with donated sperm.[19]

At this point, most physicians had little choice but to turn to commercial banks, which had the infrastructure necessary to freeze sperm, quarantine the samples, ship them, and monitor donors for months and months on end, i.e. the "assembly-line mechanisms" that had concerned Guttmacher. As small, physician-run programs at universities and private practices closed their doors and began referring patients to the large commercial banks, the total number of sperm donation programs in the United States plummeted from 139 to 28 between 1989 and 2001. Just 5 of those 28 programs had more than 90 donors, and their combined offerings constituted about half of the donors available nationwide.[20]

Indeed, founders of some of the first commercial sperm banks, which had been open but not necessarily thriving, point to AIDS as a key moment of "market expansion." The founder of Gametes Inc., which opened in 1975, described why the company's initial growth occurred at "glacial speed."

> People said the vitality, the viability of non-frozen semen is so much better than [frozen and] thawed semen. Well, yeah, duh. We could look through a microscope and see that most people's sperm didn't freeze very well, and we felt like our job is to go out and find people that had freezable sperm. We contended that our thawed sperm was just as fertile as non-frozen sperm, because we selected for really good thawed specimens. Eventually those people who were disparaging couldn't fight the utilization of frozen sperm because of the AIDS epidemic and CDC saying semen ought to be quarantined for six months. So that was a major impetus for market expansion.

Similarly, the founder of CryoCorp, which opened in 1977, sketched the growth of his company, which started out as a "one-man show."

> I found the donors, I evaluated the donors, I did the semen analysis, I did the storage, I did the freezing, I did the thawing, and I did the insemination. The clinical need for it became evident in the community, and then more and more doctors asked me to provide them with the service. With the advent of AIDS in 1984, as soon as quarantine became an accepted standard of practice, then you needed a sperm bank if you were going to provide services for infertile couples. So from there, we kept on growing and growing and growing until now we distribute about 2,500 ampules of sperm every month all over the world, and we have more donors than any of our competitors.

Given the medical profession's preference for retaining control over sperm donation, it was not happenstance that the founders of CryoCorp and Gametes Inc., one a physician and the other a PhD-trained scientist, cultivated ties to the medical establishment, maintaining appointments at local medical schools, publishing peer-reviewed articles, and giving lectures. CryoCorp's founder pointed out, "I was very academic at the time. I've written a lot about it, I lectured a lot about it, and I went to probably every hospital in [the area] discussing male infertility and sperm banking." Moreover, to this day, both banks require that a physician be involved in ordering sperm for recipients.[21] Gametes Inc.'s founder explained, "Our service is a medical product. It is well-characterized material intended for use with counseling by a physician, just like a prescription drug."[22]

The process of characterizing the material grew more elaborate over the years, as commercial banks provided additional details about donors' characteristics. CryoCorp's founder noted, "At first [patients] had one line, then one page, then two pages. Now I think the short form is three pages, and the long form could be thirty-five to fifty pages. Basically, if my wife, and I'm married thirty-eight years, read information on a donor, she would know more about the donor than she does of me." For Gametes Inc., supplying recipients with more information about donors became an explicit business strategy. The founder explained,

> We realized we could compete on technical excellence, like providing 55 million [motile sperm cells per milliliter] or more and more lab tests, but we also realized that was a sink hole, a black hole. There was always something else you could do, and the more you did, the more costly it was, not that the market could afford more. So we found it convenient to compete on a basis of providing information about our donors, and we found refuge in state regulatory authorities telling us what expectations are in terms of testing.

Such detailed information about the men producing sperm is designed to appeal to recipients, who were increasingly involved in selecting donors, another shift away from physician control that is described here by the founder of Gametes Inc.

Founder: [In the 1970s,] the principal thing was to have an inventory of freezable sperm, and we thought an inventory of ten donors was probably pretty doggone good. If you had many more than ten, the market would be just overwhelmed with choices. But it wasn't women choosing; it was physicians choosing. Later on, we got more selective with donors' physical characteristics.

Rene: When did this start to change?
Founder: In the early days, the physicians we relied on for insight into the marketplace pretty much said any donor will do. My patient

simply wants to get pregnant. It just doesn't matter who the donor is, so long as you give a Caucasian donor to a Caucasian woman and a Black donor to a Black woman. So if physicians really don't care about matching recipient and donor, ten is probably more than you really need.

Rene: So it wasn't even like they were picking the brown-haired donor or the blond donor?

Founder: I think most of the physicians we were working with were that cavalier. Some of them might look down on a catalog of ten and say you're blond and here's a blond donor. But as time went along, women probably said, "Can I see that donor catalog?" [*laughs*] And physicians said, "Yeah, sure, fifteen less seconds I have to spend with you. Take it home, and spend all the time you want."

Gametes Inc. redesigned its catalog to be "patient-friendly" in 1989, adding personal essays written by donors in 1993 and photographs of donors in 1994.

The changing demographic profile of sperm bank clientele also contributed to the demand for more information about donors. For most of the twentieth century, physicians generally limited donor insemination to heterosexual married couples. In a 1987 survey, about 50% of the physicians refused this service to unmarried heterosexual couples, and 60% refused it to single women or lesbians.[23] But in the early 1990s, a new technology called intracytoplasmic sperm injection (ICSI), in which a single sperm is injected directly into an egg cell, allowed men previously considered infertile because of low sperm count or impaired motility to forego the use of a donor. ICSI is expensive because it must be used in conjunction with IVF, but it reduced the number of heterosexual couples turning to sperm banks.

As a result, commercial banks became much more reliant on single women and lesbians, groups they had long refused to serve, and these new customers were interested in obtaining as much information about the donor as possible. Referencing his experiences with recipients over nearly four decades, CryoCorp's founder explained,

Now the recipients can't get enough information. But at that time, we weren't talking about single women, lesbian couples. We were talking about married couples, and we just tried to match the donor to the physical characteristics of the husband and left it mostly at that. But now it's mostly the single women and lesbian couples that are interested in information. When we sent the audio tapes [of donors] to a married couple, the guy would walk out of the room, because it was difficult for him to deal with the fact that his wife is being inseminated with another man's sperm.

It makes sense, then, that Western Sperm Bank was the first in the United States to offer "identity-release" donors, who agree to future contact with offspring. A nonprofit bank with roots in the feminist women's health movement, it opened in 1982 intent on serving the single women and lesbians who were barred from many university and commercial banks. With no husband to match and less investment in keeping donor insemination a secret, some of Western Sperm Bank's first customers expressed an interest in making arrangements for their children to meet the donor. To avoid legal liability for both the bank and the donor, the bank's founder decided that children could not be given identifying information about the donor until they were eighteen. Although slow to do so, many commercial banks have since followed suit.[24] Gametes Inc. began a similar program in 2001 and Cryo-Corp in 2004.

A physician who served as president of ASRM and chair of the obstetrics and gynecology department at a major research university is dismissive of all the additional information. "The bells and whistles are for the patient, not for me. What do I care if the guy is a violinist or not? It's a marketing tool. It's got nothing to do with the medicine. It has nothing to do with the quality of the sperm." He began referring patients to CryoCorp in 1991 after closing the small sperm bank at his university, because "it was an administrative problem and a legal problem, so let somebody else handle the processing of the sperm." In response to my question about whether he had provided much information about donors in his university's program, he said no, explaining "but that's the difference between a university program and a commercial program. The university asks very simple questions: eye color, height and weight, perhaps something about ethnicity. So it's going to a socialized store and a capitalist store. CryoCorp has much more information, but it's commercial, so they're selling a product. We were providing a medical service."

EGGS: THE GIFT OF LIFE

Sperm donation had been around for nearly a century by the time the first egg donation was performed, but the physicians responsible for organizing this new kind of gamete donation did not follow their own pre-existing model. They recruited donors from a different population, used different rubrics for characterizing the material, and relaxed their own requirements for anonymity between donor and recipient.

Throughout the 1970s, research teams around the world raced to be the first to claim success with *in vitro* fertilization, and the birth of Louise Brown, the first child conceived using this technique, made headlines in 1978. Although IVF with a patient's own eggs addressed some causes of infertility, such as blocked fallopian tubes, it did nothing for those without viable eggs. However, as one physician–researcher who conducted experiments with egg donation in the 1980s noted, "it doesn't take a huge leap of the imagination, if you've got dishes in the laboratory, you can get the egg from one person and put it into somebody else."

Researchers tried different techniques for doing just that, with the first pregnancies from donated eggs occurring in the mid-1980s. In one program, physicians inseminated the egg donor with sperm, waited a few days for an embryo to develop, and then flushed it out of the donor's uterus so as to implant it in the recipient. This technique is called "uterine lavage" and was first developed with cattle. But it put the egg donor at risk of sexually transmitted diseases, tubal pregnancies, and even retained pregnancies if all the embryos were not removed.[25] In another program, researchers used a different method, asking patients undergoing IVF for their own infertility to donate one of several eggs they produced to another patient. The egg was fertilized in the laboratory and then implanted in the recipient's uterus.[26] By the late 1980s, a new technique for retrieving eggs reduced the level of risk associated with this outpatient procedure and made it acceptable to ask women who were not already undergoing fertility treatments to serve as egg donors.[27]

To find egg donors, physicians looked not to students in need of extra cash but to women in the surrounding community. Describing how the "initial cohort of donors" was recruited for the uterine flushing experiments, a physician–researcher recalled,

> They put an advertisement in the paper saying: "Help an infertile woman have a baby. We are looking for women who have completed childbearing who previously were extremely fertile." So they recruited a cohort, and I want to say that they screened a hundred women and got twenty of them. And they were paid very little, I want to say $500, and imagine what they had to go through. The idea was that they would have all of these women, all similar looking, and they had a set of recipients that would simply say, "Well, I'll take any one of these." In talking to the investigators at the time, they called them Earth Mothers. These women were really into the whole motherhood experience.

As more universities around the country began offering IVF and recruiting egg donors, their advertisements also incorporated maternal imagery and called on women to "help" others. Montefiore Medical Center placed the following radio ad in 1992, "A Westchester fertility center is seeking altruistic and compassionate women under thirty-six years of age who are willing to donate their eggs to women who are unable to have children because of lack of eggs. Financial compensation is available."[28] Clinicians at the University of California–Irvine published a study in 1993 that pointed out "volunteers are women from the community surrounding the medical center . . . A periodic advertisement has been placed in a major metropolitan newspaper on a prominent page. It pictures a mother and a baby and asks if the reader is a woman under thirty-five who would like to help an infertile woman to have a child through egg donation."[29]

In appealing to women's sense of altruism, physicians placed much more emphasis on egg donors' motivations than they ever had with sperm donors. In fact, the earliest egg donation programs incorporated psychological evaluations, in part to assess women's motivations, a form of screening that had rarely, if ever, been required of men donating sperm.[30]

But, as Cleveland Clinic researchers reasoned in a 1989 article, they needed to make sure that women were motivated by something more than money because "financial gain as a primary motive seems to be a negative prognostic indicator for compliance with the program."[31] Twenty years later, Eric Surrey, past president of the Society for Assisted Reproductive Technology (SART), expressed identical sentiments in an interview with Reuters reporters. "We understand that financial compensation is certainly one motivation, but should never be the sole motivation. These women are providing a great gift to others that should not be taken lightly."[32]

Indeed, in talking with a physician–researcher about the early days of egg donation, he underscored the importance of women's motivations before mentioning their medical history in describing the screening he does.

Physician: Screening for people who are motivated properly, motivated because they want to help somebody, not just because they need money. That's a real issue. Screen them psychologically, make sure they're healthy, infectious diseases, family history to make sure they have no genetic diseases.

Rene: *You're transferring biological tissue, so I can certainly understand why you would want to do all the medical screening, but why did it matter what their motivations were?*
Physician: Well, because if their motivation isn't correct, then they may not be telling you the truth. Their motivation, it may cloud their honesty in terms of saying whether they have had an infectious disease in the past or whether there's a genetic disease in the family. That's always concerned recipients: how much can you rely on what the donor says? Because there's no independent verification of what the donor gives you in terms of the history. So that's one of the main reasons you'd like them to be properly motivated. Also they have to do things exactly right. So if they're really well motivated and have the best interests of the recipient in mind, they're altruistic, they're less likely to screw up on medications or something that they should be doing.

In providing a rationale for the expectation that women have altruistic motivations, this physician uses altruism as a proxy for honesty about medical information, which, as he notes, there is no way of verifying.

This is also true of sperm donors' medical history, but there is no such expectation that men be altruistically motivated. In fact, the 2006 edition of the ASRM patient guide *Third Party Reproduction* recommends that egg donors be evaluated for their motivations but contains no analogous recommendation for sperm donors.

Physicians also deviated from the sperm donor model in that they were less insistent on strict anonymity between donor and recipient. At the University of Southern California, one of the first programs to offer egg donation, a full quarter of the first 325 cycles, which took place between 1987 and 1993, involved donors whom recipients had brought into the program.[33] A survey of other early egg donation programs revealed that more than half required recipients to bring in their own donors.[34] As a study published in *Fertility and Sterility* in 1995 noted, "Ovum donation evolved differently from sperm donation. The first case of ovum donation used an anonymous donor, but, in subsequent clinical practice, known donors, such as a sister or friend, became common. It was the advent of ovum donation that began to raise questions about the assumptions that had traditionally accompanied donor insemination."[35]

Another contrast with sperm donation is that, to this day, egg donation usually involves fresh eggs. It is possible to freeze sperm and to freeze embryos, but freezing eggs is still in the experimental stages, primarily because of the high water content in these large cells.[36] Although the exact levels of risk of transmitting particular diseases via eggs are not clear, egg donors are fully screened for a range of sexually transmitted diseases.

The trajectory of egg donation did mimic that of sperm donation in one crucial way: the medical profession eventually had to cede control of egg donor recruitment to commercial agencies, a process driven by rapidly increasing recipient demand. As one physician–researcher explained, in the early days, it was not clear how many people would need donated eggs.

> In 1984, egg donation was a speck on the horizon, a gee-whiz, but really how applicable is this going to be? Sperm donation seemed much more obvious. Lots of men didn't have sperm, but women, as near as we could

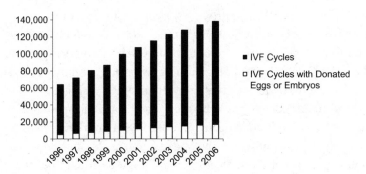

Figure 1. Proportion of IVF cycles involving donated eggs or embryos, by year

tell, all had eggs, except for the rare few who had premature ovarian failure, meaning menopause under the age of 35. We thought they would be the only potential recipients, and that was indeed the first group. We thought older women were not going to get pregnant no matter what you did to them. It was serendipity that some of the women with premature ovarian failure had turned 40 by the time we got our program going. When we did egg donation to them, lo and behold, they got pregnant at very high rates, at the same rates as the young women. And it was like, "Oh, oh, it's in the egg. The older uterus is not a problem." This is obvious now, but this was the big a-ha moment.[37]

Up until the early 1990s, most physicians had very little experience providing IVF with egg donation; one survey revealed that just 10% of fertility clinics had performed more than ten cycles in the previous two years.[38] However, by the time the CDC started tabulating statistics on IVF in 1996, there were more than 300 fertility clinics in the United States, 74% of which offered egg donation. Over the next decade, the number of IVF cycles performed in the United States rose steadily, from around 64,000 per year to nearly 140,000 in 2006, with the proportion of those involving donated eggs or embryos growing from 8% to 12% (see Figure 1).[39]

As IVF with donated eggs became more popular, especially among older women, physicians had trouble keeping up with the demand. The first commercial egg agencies opened their doors around 1990, offering rosters of women willing to provide sex cells in return for financial compensation. One of the earliest programs, and now one of the largest in the country, OvaCorp, emerged out of an established surrogacy agency on the West Coast. A psychologist there, who had already been screening surrogate mothers and matching them with recipients for several years, described receiving two phone calls around the same time in the late 1980s. One woman had been diagnosed with premature ovarian failure, and she called saying, "I don't need a uterus. My uterus works fine. Do you think any of the women who are volunteering to be surrogates would volunteer just to give me their eggs?" The psychologist replied that she did not know and promised to get back to her. After talking with the agency's owners, she decided to ask a few women who had previously served as surrogates. She explained, "They'd already given up a whole baby, so giving up an egg seemed relatively easy." The second call came from a woman who said, "I'd really like to help someone, but I hate being pregnant. Is there anything I could do? I waste eggs every month." As in the physician's description of one of the first egg donations in a medical setting, the gendered tropes of giving and helping also appear in this narrative of one of the first egg donations in a commercial setting.

In explaining the significance of these two calls, the psychologist pointed out that "egg donation was certainly going on. It wasn't like we had never heard of it, but the idea that we would be involved had not ever dawned on us." But compared to surrogacy, which had been so controversial, egg donation "was a piece of cake," and "pretty soon [the agency's owners] understood that this was going to be something. They started advertising for donors and letting doctors know that we were doing it."

Women who donated eggs in the early 1990s were paid between $500 and $3,500 per cycle.[40] In deciding how much to pay egg donors, one physician–researcher said he set the fee based on a "gut reaction to what would be reasonable." Others were more systematic. The Cleveland Clinic assigned economic value to each stage of the donation cycle, paying women $50 for each day they received injected hormones or had blood drawn; $100 for days when they received injected hormones, had blood drawn, *and* had an ultrasound; and $350 for the day of egg retrieval. This usually resulted in a total payment of $900 to $1,200 per cycle.[41]

Similarly, the psychologist at OvaCorp said she "sat down and really calculated how many appointments" donors attended, because she believed that "women's time was worth something."

> We decided $2,500, based on the fact that surrogates got 10 or 12 [thousand dollars] for fifteen months of work [in the late 1980s]. A donor was going to have to commit for three months by the time they did five intakes, injections, their pain and suffering physically. Nothing compares to labor I guess, but it was uncomfortable. Also, we wanted it to be an amount of money that was respectful, but not enticing. They get the money whether there is a pregnancy or not, so you wanted women to do it because they were going to do a good job, not just because they were dirt poor. It felt right. No one argued with that fee. The doctors weren't uncomfortable. The couples weren't uncomfortable.

The founder of what is today another major egg agency on the West Coast noted that when she opened in 1991, $2,500 was the "going rate," so that is what she paid donors.

In figuring out how to recruit egg donors and match them with recipients, OvaCorp also did not look to sperm donation as a model. The psychologist explained, "We came from the adoption world and the surrogacy world, not the sperm donor medical world and organ donor world. So we just did it from a very informed consent, patient advocacy, you've-all-agreed-prior-to-conception, all-cards-on-the-table perspective versus let's micromanage information and the doctor-will-have-the-only-copy model." Committed to the open flow of information between donor and recipient, she did not *allow* anonymity, requiring that both parties meet one another. She explained the process.

> I would meet with the parents to narrow down what they were looking for. I would present them with a couple of choices, not a catalog. The couples were not obsessively picky, because that wasn't the market at the time. There weren't twenty [egg] agencies to go to. Then I would set up a meeting with the recipients and the donor at my office. We'd sit and talk for an hour and a half. If they liked each other, then the attorney would draft a contract. We would send them to the IVF clinic, and they'd be on their way.

Although the process of characterizing the material happened very differently in the first commercial egg agencies than it had in the sperm banks, information about the donors was deemed similarly powerful in attracting customers. According to the psychologist, OvaCorp was soon hearing from recipients all over the world.

> . . . If [the recipients] wanted to know more, have control, wanted a specific type of genetic history, Chinese, Jewish, harder-to-find donors. If they lived in a small town and knew the [egg] donors were the two nurses downstairs, that was too weird. If a couple was from overseas and the waiting list was really long, they'd come to us, and we'd match them with a choice of donors within a few months. That's no big deal now, but it was a big deal in 1990 because there was the idea of choice, the idea of information.

In fact, one of OvaCorp's first clients was a couple from New York whose university donation program did not have any African American donors. OvaCorp's psychologist recalled, "They called me, and I said 'Sure; her name is Michelle. When would you like to meet her?' I only had a few, but I had them. So they came all the way to California, paid handsomely for it, instead of doing it right in New York."

Indeed, the situation was very different on the two coasts. Commercial egg agencies did not open in the East for several years, and a West Coast physician–researcher describes a similar situation in the 1990s, when he had "patients coming from New York, because they were much slower in developing egg donation and good numbers of egg donors." To this day, physician-run programs in the East are more insistent on anonymity and reveal less information about egg donors. The founder of the second egg agency to open on the West Coast explained that "the main difference was not showing pictures [of donors]. People didn't believe, and still don't believe, that an egg donation needs to involve a photograph. The doctors can control that. We get those calls all the time."

Given their proximity to the nascent commercial egg agencies, doctors on the West Coast began to adopt similarly open policies. One physician–researcher described how, as was standard practice in sperm donation, "initially, we were matching [egg donors and recipients]. Then gradually we got wind of the fact that other places were showing people pictures, and we had a big debate about whether we would show pictures. We decided that that would really demystify it, so we started showing pictures." These kinds of innovations eventually made their way back to sperm banks, evident in Gametes Inc.'s and CryoCorp's decisions to start providing additional information about sperm donors in the 1990s. However, while some sperm banks offer baby photos of donors, many, including CryoCorp, still do not provide adult photos and most do not allow meetings between sperm donors and recipients.

OvaCorp's first major competitor, founded by a therapist who herself had undergone treatment for infertility, opened in 1991. When asked how she went from patient to broker, she also referenced the importance of information.

> There were sperm donor programs and surrogacy programs, but there wasn't an organized way of finding egg donors. Other than OvaCorp, there really wasn't anybody saying we have a roster of women, here's information about them. I went up to my doctor and said "I think I can help you. I think I can recruit egg donors." I knew there was a need, and doctors are really busy, so if you take a burden off their shoulders, they're thrilled [*laughs*]. He said absolutely, because he knew me. I went around knocking on other doctors' offices, but only one really got behind the idea. He was wonderfully supportive, started referring me patients, and we did a number of donations together. The other doctors were real closed about it. Two years later, I began to have success and became known in the industry, and of course they were calling me: "Why aren't you working with us?"

Indeed, some egg agencies receive enough inquiries from patients to serve as an important referral source for physicians, with one founder noting that it can "make you really powerful."

Although OvaCorp required that egg donors have children of their own, the new program did not, and the founder also focused her recruitment efforts on the local entertainment industry. She explained that, in the early 1990s, it was not obvious where to find donors.

> Back then, no one knew what [egg donation] was. I had been an actress. I thought, actresses have time off, they're attractive, and they're usually

fairly bright. I ran an ad in [an acting newspaper] saying, "extremely re-warding emotionally and financially, become an egg donor." I had about 75 calls for the first ad, and it went from there.

It was around this time that OvaCorp's psychologist was "having lunch with a very well-known IVF doctor. He said, 'you better take note, that new agency is going to be really great. Their donors are models and ac-tresses and really high quality. You got competition.'" Indeed, as the num-ber of commercial egg agencies began to grow, many allowed women without children to become donors, and OvaCorp was forced to change its policies "to compete." Once it did so, the psychologist explained, "of course, OvaCorp had hundreds more donors."

In the early 1990s, there were just a few commercial agencies, but by the end of the decade, one program director described them as "escalating exponentially. It's insane how much competition there is."[42] One of the new agencies, Creative Beginnings, was founded in 1999 by a nurse who had worked in fertility practices for years, including a period in which she managed a prominent physician–researcher's egg donation pro-gram. Like several other women with this background, she decided to strike out on her own, explaining "I have a reputation for starting [this physician's] donor program, co-authoring research with him. Doctors tell me they're really happy to see me doing this, that I come from the right background." When she was working for physicians, she explained,

> I would get donors from all these different [agencies] that were not in-formed, didn't know what they were getting into, and I had donors I couldn't get a hold of. The nurses have to educate them, make sure they do this right, and if they don't, it's the nurses' fault. I didn't have very much power. And then I saw they were totally inappropriate when I'd read their medical history.

It was for these reasons that the founder of Creative Beginnings thought of herself as the "right person" to open a commercial egg agency.

Whereas compensation to sperm donors had rarely generated much debate, questions about whether and how much to pay women for pro-viding eggs were raised early and often, including in editorial exchanges in the *New England Journal of Medicine* in 1993 and *Fertility and Sterility* in

1999.[43] This latter exchange was sparked by a New York donation program's decision to raise donor fees in 1998, in the words of the editorial writer, "to double the compensation from the community standard of $2,500 to a startling $5,000 per cycle." Indeed, the price hike was covered on the front page of the *New York Times*.[44] The physician responsible for the increase justified it on the grounds that he had a six-month waiting list for recipients, noting that most clinics were experiencing "very strong demand" for egg donors. Yet this $5,000 figure, which seemed shocking at the time, was deemed acceptable just a year later in an ASRM ethics statement, which concluded that sums above $5,000 "require justification and sums above $10,000 are not appropriate."[45]

Throughout the 2000s, ASRM persisted in drawing a line at $5,000, but egg donor fees continued to rise. Several physician–researchers blamed commercial agencies, as in this 2006 interview with a past president of SART.

> With the involvement of agencies, the payment of the donors has crept up to a level that makes physicians a little bit uncomfortable. The whole question is whether at some point it becomes coercive. A person decides to do egg donation partly because of the money, and that kind of coerces them into accepting the risks of egg donation. We would have liked to see it stay down in the 3, 4, 5,000 [dollar] range where it's more just compensating them for their time, their effort, to some extent the risks that they go under, discomforts. Everyone could have a different opinion on that, but I think that when it gets up to levels like 7,000 [dollars], it's more than just compensating the patient for those other things.

In an attempt to rein in fees, SART's executive committee sent a letter to egg agencies in 2006 informing them of the expectation that they abide by the ASRM guidelines. Egg donation programs that agreed in writing were then included on a list of "approved agencies," which was posted on SART's and ASRM's websites. However, as professional societies, these organizations do not have any regulatory power to enforce limits on compensation, and they do not independently verify the actual fees paid to donors.[46] The debate over compensating women for eggs continues to the present day, with articles appearing on the front page of *USA Today* and in the *New York Times*.[47]

As in sperm donation, physicians resisted the shift to commercial egg agencies, because they would have preferred to continue recruiting their own donors. One physician–researcher, who was among the first to offer egg donation in the United States, described the state of affairs in the mid-2000s, echoing Titmuss and Guttmacher in assuming that pecuniary motives are incompatible with ethical practices.

> We have now a situation that I think is not very good, where the egg donor agencies sort of out-hustle and out-advertise the IVF programs. We no longer have our own donors [in my university program], except maybe three or four that came in by word of mouth, but we no longer advertise. The agencies really jacked up the price, and they have an entirely different mindset. We were trying to get recipients pregnant. We wanted to make sure we had the best kind of donor that we possibly could have, and of course we wanted to make sure we protected the donors. The agency is motivated to sell the donor, so they want the donor to be attractive and appear as good as possible, not so much to screen them out. We get recipients who are already very much invested in a particular donor. We then find out the donor lives in [another state], is not available, wants to come down and do as little as possible. The agency is putting pressure on us saying "This donor is very reliable, blah, blah, blah, everything should be good." And so we're [hormonally] stimulating somebody that we're not watching. There's clearly been a shift in the way that these things are being done. Yes, another doctor can see her there, but is somebody holding her hand? Is somebody actually asking her whether she's having issues with injections? You get a lot more information from a patient-doctor interaction than just looking at a piece of paper that has ultrasound. And the donors go from program to program, and the doctor doesn't have experience as to how they responded [to the medications] last time. Previously the donor was with us; by the third or fourth time, it was autopilot.

When asked how he would organize egg donation if he had the only program in the country, he harkened back to an earlier era of physician control, saying "I would go back to the way we used to really have personal hands-on control over all of the egg donors."

It is striking that OvaCorp's psychologist expresses similar concerns about the "business people" running egg agencies. Here, she described OvaCorp's initial pitch to physicians at fertility practices in the early 1990s.

We used to say to the doctors that they're really trained in medicine, but once they became brokers, they were really working out of their expertise and having staff do things they weren't trained for. Why not say to the patients, "Listen, I'm the doctor; I have certain requirements. Here's ten agencies: Get your donor, get her screened, let them hold your hand, do your legal, and then come back when you're ready." So much cleaner, really. The upside is the doctors stopped making their offices so labor heavy with all the hysterics of egg donation, and it gave couples a lot more choice and freedom and access. On the downside, it turned egg donation out of the hands of professional, licensed people who are accountable to a higher level, meaning AMA [the American Medical Association], and turned it over to people who don't have any professional liability, any code of ethics. They're just business people, not accountable to anybody. If you want to change an egg donor application to make it look better, if you want to erase the word alcoholism or whatever, there's nothing stopping you.

For just these reasons, several physicians underscored the importance of vigilance when it comes to referring patients to egg agencies, especially given the lack of regulation in this market. One said, "The most important thing is to recognize they're not all equal, and so individual practices should be sure that an agency is doing a good, thorough job." Another noted that his practice only refers to agencies where "we know the people that run them personally, know them to be responsible, and we have not had bad experiences with the donors."

ONE OF THE HOLDOUTS

While most physicians turned to commercial providers for sex cells, some continue to maintain their own small sperm and egg donation programs. University Fertility Services falls into this category, and in 2006, the medical director there referenced the importance of physician control in describing his rationale for running a small bank, which included samples from just ten sperm donors.[48]

We knew our donors, so not only on paper do they pass everything, but we had a relationship with them and believe in their honesty when they said, 'No, I haven't had any more sexual partners in the last six months.' Rather than I've got something from [CryoCorp] that lists those things, and, well, I hope that's all true. That was the big difference from our standpoint. We just had a better feeling that we knew these donors and had control over it.

However, given the small size of their donor pool, University Fertility Services also finds it necessary to refer patients to CryoCorp and Gametes Inc.

As a result of impending FDA regulations, the university decided to stop recruiting sperm donors in 2001. The embryologist there explained,

To maintain a [sperm] donor program is time- and employee-intensive, and since there are other agencies that can provide that type of thing, it is probably becoming less available within a particular program. A university program is not just doing IVF and donor; they're doing all sorts of other things as well. The medical director [here] has wanted to provide full-service everything, and I think we've done a pretty good job of that until the FDA came through [laughs]. It just burdened us down personnel-wise and added time and expense that, as a smaller program, we couldn't see our way through to extending that cost and personnel time for a condition that we could make use of elsewhere. And the patient's gonna pay for it one way or another [laughs].

At the same time, University Fertility Services continues to recruit egg donors, even though the medical director described it as a "hassle." He said, "With egg donors, there is no bank that you order from and it comes in the mail. Essentially, you either have your own donors, or you send your patients away to another program. So we go through all the hassle of recruiting and screening." A review of the university's charts reveals that a total of 149 women signed up to donate eggs between 1993 and 2005. However, it appears that only about half completed a cycle: 30% of the women donated once, 13% donated twice, 8% donated three times, and 2% donated between four and six times.

The founder of Gametes Inc. also pointed to the importance of monetary motivations in explaining why some physicians continue to recruit their own egg donors.

Surgeons consume blood, but they aren't responsible for finding blood donors. Somebody else does that for the surgeons. So the physicians practicing reproductive medicine probably didn't need to be out looking for gamete donors. The fact of the matter is that some of them think that that's an important part of their practice, and I suspect that some of their personnel encouraged their doctors to think that way, because that's how their salary is justified, that they evaluate egg donors. I don't think any of these people, or very few of these people any more, bother to seek out sperm donors. But there is still a substantial number that recruit and evaluate egg donors for their patients. And it's remunerative for them. They not only recover their cost, there's value added on top of that. We think as time goes along physicians in reproductive medicine will pass on that responsibility to others. We think they'll be encouraged to do that in part by regulation.

Like other physicians, the medical director at University Fertility Services expressed skepticism about commercial egg agencies, saying it was they who "need to be regulated." In particular, he raised questions about the expertise of their personnel and the high prices paid to donors. Like other academic programs, University Fertility Services offers less compensation than commercial agencies; egg donors received just $2,000 per cycle in 2006. As a holdout in a world where the going rate is $5,000, the nurses and physicians in the practice lament the difficulty they have in recruiting enough women to provide eggs for their patients.[49]

Ironically, one effect of drawing the line at too much commodification is that University Fertility Services sometimes had to be less choosy than commercial agencies. For example, in one session I observed there, the psychologist was screening a prospective egg donor, whom she later described to me as completely unacceptable. The applicant's financial situation seemed precarious, she did not like the idea of taking hormones, and she did not seem to understand that she would need to take hormones for several weeks to stimulate egg production. However, the nurse–coordinator wanted the applicant to continue with the screening process, because there was a list of recipients who had been waiting months for a donor. This episode suggests that there are not always obvious lines to be drawn in the market for sex cells and that the drive to generate revenue leads to complicated calculations by commercial and university donation programs alike.[50]

CONCLUSION

As scientific experiments in assisted reproduction became standard clinical practice, both sperm and egg donation traveled the path from medical service to commercial good. In outsourcing the procurement of sperm and eggs, physicians reflected broader trends in medicine during the last third of the twentieth century, including challenges to their professional authority, which came in part from newly constituted patient- and consumer-rights groups, several of which were part of the broader women's health movement. The medical profession was also contending with explosive growth in the health care sector of the U.S. economy.[51] In 1980, Arnold Relman, then editor of the *New England Journal of Medicine*, dubbed it a "medical–industrial complex," describing a "large and growing network of private corporations engaged in the business of supplying health-care services to patients for a profit—services heretofore provided by nonprofit institutions or individual practitioners."[52] This description certainly encompasses the commercial sperm banks and egg agencies that came into existence around this time.

To procure sperm, commercial banks that first opened in the 1970s largely mimicked the physicians they sought to supplant, recruiting students, prioritizing high sperm count, and offering a range of physiognomies to match recipients' husbands. It was not until the demographics of their clientele began to change to include more single women and lesbian couples that commercial banks began expanding their efforts to provide more information about sperm donors. At the same time, banks were responding to a more general trend of patients demanding more control over their medical care. But the egg donation programs that emerged in the 1980s and 1990s did not adopt the already-established model of gamete donation provided by sperm donation. Emphasizing altruistic motivations, programs recruited caring women from the broader community who wanted to help infertile couples have a child, and they allowed, and in some cases even encouraged, donors and recipients to meet.

In characterizing the reproductive material on offer, donation programs used a similar strategy to personify sperm and eggs: the provision of ever-more extensive information about the donors. However, the kinds of information deemed important depend on whether the person donating is a man or a woman. Program staff emphasize different aspects of who egg and sperm donors are, their personalities and characteristics, and they share different types of information with sperm recipients and egg recipients. The next chapter offers a detailed look inside contemporary sperm banks and egg agencies, and it reveals how these initial patterns, driven by beliefs about biological sex differences and gendered expectations of donors, calcified into countless organizational processes, suffusing the medical market for sex cells.

TWO Selling Genes, Selling Gender

Contemporary egg agencies and sperm banks operate within the context of a thriving medical marketplace. In many cases, the programs are founded or staffed by physicians, nurses, and psychologists. They cultivate networks with referring physicians, belong to professional medical associations, set goals for expanding their businesses, charge a variety of fees for different services, and develop official protocols for dealing with donors and recipients. Even when the donation program staff members are not actually clinicians, they are part of the broader medical market for sex cells and, as such, are able to draw on the cultural power of medical authority in shaping the structure and meaning of egg and sperm donation.[1]

To stay in business, donation programs must recruit "sellable" donors who provide "high-quality" gametes to recipients who "shop around."

In the words of OvaCorp's psychologist, "Medically, the invention of IVF really broke it down to [fallopian] tubes, eggs, uterus, sperm. To this day, that's how we solve the problem. Do you need sperm or eggs, or do you need both? Or do you need a uterus? What do you got, what do you need, and what can you give up psychologically? Then sort of broker what you need." But even as egg agencies and sperm banks engage in similar practices—advertising to recruit donors, screening applicants, monitoring the production of bodily goods, and setting fees—a detailed comparison of their organizational processes reveals that what makes an egg donor sellable is not what makes a sperm donor sellable and that the definition of "high quality" is not the same for women and men.

This chapter details the daily business practices of two egg agencies, OvaCorp and Creative Beginnings, and two sperm banks, CryoCorp and Western Sperm Bank. Economic rhetoric permeates all four programs, but staff members are very aware of being in a unique business. They discuss "people-management" strategies and point out that they are not "manufacturing toothpaste" or "selling pens." They also consistently refer to the women and men who produce eggs and sperm as "donors" who "help" recipients, and they refer to the donor-recipient exchange as a "win-win situation." But as will become clear, cultural beliefs about sex and gender shape this confluence of economic logic and altruistic rhetoric so that in egg agencies donation means giving a gift while in sperm banks it means performing a job. To assess whether these differences persist even in programs that sell both eggs and sperm, where one might expect such distinctions to be more apparent, I conclude the chapter with a brief discussion of Gametes Inc. and University Fertility Services.

RECRUITING "SELLABLE" DONORS

To find donors, egg agencies and sperm banks advertise in a variety of forums (college newspapers, free weekly magazines, radio, and websites), hold donor information sessions, and encourage previous donors to refer siblings, friends, and roommates. CryoCorp and Western Sperm Bank are located within blocks of prestigious four-year universities, and their

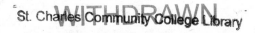

advertising is directed at cash-strapped college students. The marketing director of CryoCorp, which requires that donors be enrolled in or have a degree from a four-year university, explained that the location was a deliberate choice because "the owners of the sperm bank thought that that was a good job match, and it really works out well for the students. They're young and therefore healthy. They don't have to make a huge time commitment. They can visit the sperm bank anytime." Nevertheless, the staff members at sperm banks lament difficulties in recruiting men and offer hefty "finder's fees" to current donors who refer successful applicants.

In contrast, OvaCorp and Creative Beginnings receive several hundred applications from women each month. Creative Beginnings' founder explained the impetus behind her marketing strategy. "We appeal to the idea that there's an emotional reward, that they're going to feel good about what they've done, that it's a win-win situation, that they're going to help someone with something that person needs, and they're going to get something they need in return." Both agencies report that "young moms are the best donors. They pay the best attention and show up for appointments" because they understand the importance of a child to recipient clients.

When a potential donor calls or e-mails a program for the first time, the staff initiates an extensive screening process by asking about family health history (including physical, mental, and genetic disease) and social characteristics. Some screening standards are based on biomedical guidelines for genetic material most likely to result in pregnancy. For example, ASRM issues guidelines for age and height/weight ratios, which are followed closely by egg agencies to select donors who will respond well to fertility medications. But some of the guidelines reflect recipient requests for socially desirable characteristics, such as the height minimums set by sperm banks at around 5 feet 8 inches.

Even some of the nominally biomedical factors are better understood as social characteristics, as evident in this donor manager's discussion of Western Sperm Bank's standards.

> We have to not take people that are very overweight because of a sellable issue. It becomes a marketing thing; some of the people we don't accept.

Also height becomes a marketing thing. When I'm interviewing somebody to be a donor, of course personality is really important. Are they
gonna be responsible? But immediately I'm also clicking in my mind: Are
they blond? Are they blue-eyed? Are they tall? Are they Jewish? So [I'm]
not just looking at the [sperm] counts and the [health] history but also can
we sell this donor? And anyone that's [willing to release identifying information to offspring at age eighteen], obviously we will ignore a lot;
even if they're not quite as tall as we'd like, we'll take them. Or maybe if
they're a little chunky, we'll still take them, because we know that [their
willingness to release identifying information] will supersede the other
stuff.

Likewise, in explaining the screening process for women applying to be
donors, Creative Beginnings' office manager said, "this is a business, and
we're trying to provide a service." Later that day, her assistant noted that
recipients "basically go shopping and they want this and they want that."

OvaCorp's donor manager also emphasized social characteristics, including education level and attractiveness, in describing what makes an
egg donor "sellable."

You will find that a donor's selling tool is her brains and her beauty. That's
a donor's selling point, as opposed to she's a wonderful person. That's
nice. But bottom line, everyone wants someone that's either very attractive, someone very healthy, and someone very bright. That's her selling
point/tool. That's why I also work with women who don't have children,
because I get a higher level of academia with a lot of our single donors
because they're not distracted by kids.

Research on how recipients select donors suggests that staff members
are responding to their clients' interest in attractive and intelligent donors whose phenotypes are similar to their own.[2] Egg agencies and
sperm banks use education as a signifier of genetic-based intelligence,
but as the donor manager quoted above suggests, women without children have more time to pursue additional schooling.[3]

During this early phase of recruitment, egg agency staff members are
also assessing an applicant's level of responsibility, which is often glossed
as "personality" or "helpfulness," as in this interview with the assistant
director of Creative Beginnings.

Assistant Director: Personality is a big thing. We always want this to be a positive experience, if it is going to bring them to a different point in their life instead of just doing it to do it. A lot of them don't care about the money; they just want to help somebody, and that's all the more reason to continue with them.

Rene: So if donors don't ever meet the recipient, though, why would their personality matter technically?
Assistant Director: Well, we don't really look at the personality for them to meet the recipient. If they have a good personality, then we can trust them. They really want to go forward with this. They're more likely to continue with the process by getting their profile finished in a timely manner, getting their pictures into us and all the release forms that they need. Then it just shows responsibility.

At the same time, according to Creative Beginnings' founder, the staff is responding to recipients who "want to know that the person donating is a good person. They want to know that person wasn't doing it for the money, that person's family history is good, that person was reasonably smart, that they weren't fly-by-nights, drug abusers, or prostitutes." Intersecting with gendered expectations about egg donors having, or at least expressing, altruistic motivations are class-based concerns around defining "appropriate" donors.

Sperm banks, in stark contrast, *expect* men to be financially motivated, and the staff speaks directly about responsibility rather than couching it in terms of altruistic motivations. Western Sperm Bank's donor manager explained,

> Aside from personality, the other thing that makes me fall in love with a donor is someone that's responsible. It is so rare to get someone that's truly responsible, that comes in when he's supposed to come in or at least has the courtesy to call us and say, "I can't make it this week, but I'll come in next week twice." Then of course the second thing that makes him ideal is that he has consistently very high [sperm] counts, so I rarely have to toss anything on him [i.e., reject his sperm sample]. And then, I guess the third thing would be someone that has a great personality, that's just adorable, caring, and sweet. There are donors, that their personalities, I

think, ugh. They have great [sperm] counts, they come in when they're supposed to, but I just don't like them. That's a personal thing, and I think, huh, I don't want more of those babies out in the world.

Although egg agencies and sperm banks are interested in responsible women and men who fulfill their obligations, donors are also expected to embody notions of American femininity or masculinity. Staff members expect egg donors to conform to one of two gendered stereotypes: highly educated and physically attractive or caring and motherly with children of their own. Sperm donors, on the other hand, are generally expected to be tall and college educated with consistently high sperm counts.

In terms of other characteristics, egg agencies and sperm banks work to recruit donors from a variety of racial, ethnic, and religious backgrounds to satisfy a diverse recipient population. In fact, race/ethnicity is genetically reified to the degree that it serves as the basis for program filing systems. In Creative Beginnings' office, there is a cabinet for "active donor" files. The top two drawers are labeled "Caucasian," and the bottom drawer is labeled "Black, Asian, Hispanic." During a tour of Cryo-Corp, the founder lifted sperm samples out of the storage tank filled with liquid nitrogen and explained that the vials are capped with white tops for Caucasian donors, black tops for African American donors, yellow tops for Asian donors, and red tops for donors with "mixed ancestry." All four programs complain about the difficulty of recruiting African American, Hispanic, and Asian donors, and Jewish donors are in demand for Jewish clients. In one case, even though a director thought a particular egg donor applicant was too interested in the financial compensation, she was accepted into the program because she was Catholic, reflecting the director's interest in diversifying the donor catalog.

The final phase of recruitment involves reproductive endocrinologists, psychologists, and geneticists or genetic counselors, who serve as professional stamps of approval in producing sex cells for sale.[4] Applicants are examined by a physician and tested for blood type, Rh factor, drugs, and sexually transmitted infections. Both egg agencies require a psychological evaluation and the Minnesota Multiphasic Personality Inventory, but neither sperm bank requires that donors be psychologically screened. All four programs require that donors prepare a detailed family health history for three generations (and thus do not generally accept adoptees). In some programs, this history is evaluated by genetic counselors or geneticists, who might request specific genetic tests. In at least one case, though, test results revealing the mutation that causes cystic fibrosis were not enough to disqualify an "extraordinary" egg donor. The founder of Creative Beginnings explained,

> All the time there are calls coming in about problems or questions. Like today, there is a donor who's mixed. She's got Black and Caucasian, and her cystic fibrosis screening turned out that she's a carrier.[5] She's a really pretty girl, and the recipient really wants her badly because she's fair skinned, she's very pretty, and the recipient knows that this donor is extraordinary. But then [the recipient is] torn because her husband's saying, "Well, do we want to introduce something into our gene pool?" They could go ahead and use her, but the husband just has to be tested to see if he's a carrier.

As part of describing why she is the "right person" to open a commercial egg agency (discussed in Chapter 1), the founder of Creative Beginnings criticized other programs for just this scenario, which underscores the difficulty of refusing paying clients who become attached to a particular donor.

Staff members at each of the four programs view donor screening as a staged process that requires more of a monetary investment at every step. According to one of OvaCorp's psychologists, the psychological screening in egg donation is often performed before the medical tests because it is cheaper. Similarly, in sperm donation, banks confirm that a donor passes one set of tests before advancing him because, according to a Western Sperm Bank donor screener, "at each step of the game, we're spending more money on them." CryoCorp's marketing director takes this rationale a step further: "Once someone goes through our screening process, it's in our best interest to continue him in the program, because we've invested a huge amount of money, thousands and thousands of dollars. So the more vials we can collect before he drops out of the program, the better, especially if that donor's a popular donor."

In this first stage in the process of gamete donation, there are structural similarities in that both egg agencies and sperm banks expend funds on recruitment and employ a range of medical and social standards to garner "sellable" donors. But comparing how staff evaluates donors and their genetic material reveals how gendered stereotypes shape the definition of "high-quality" eggs and sperm. Both women and men are screened for infectious and genetic diseases, which suggests parallel concerns raised by the exchange of bodily tissue. However, "girls who just want to lay their eggs for some quick cash" are rejected, while men are expected to be interested in making money.

These gendered expectations correspond to traditional norms of women as selfless caregivers and men as emotionally distant breadwinners, a link between individual reproductive cells and cultural norms of motherhood and fatherhood that is made especially clear in the psychological evaluations, which are required of egg donors but not sperm donors. In addition to being evaluated for psychological stability, women are asked how they feel about "having their genetics out there." Sperm banks do not require that men consider this question with a mental health professional, which suggests that women are perceived as more closely connected to their eggs than men are to their sperm.

The majority of women and men who apply to donation programs are not accepted. Both sperm banks reject more than 90% of applicants, most because they do not have the exceptionally high sperm counts that are required because freezing sperm in liquid nitrogen significantly reduces the number that are motile. Both egg agencies estimate that they reject over 80% of women who apply.[6] In short, donor recruitment is time intensive, rigorous, and costly. As staff members sift through hundreds of applications, the framing of egg donation as an altruistic win-win situation and sperm donation as an easy job shapes subsequent staff/donor interactions, from constructing individualized donor profiles to the actual sale of sex cells.

CONSTRUCTING DONOR PROFILES

Once applicants pass the initial screening with program staff, they are invited to fill out a "donor profile." These are lengthy documents with questions about the donor's physical characteristics, family health history, and educational attainment; in some programs, standardized test scores, GPA, and IQ scores are requested. There are also open-ended questions about hobbies, likes and dislikes, and motivations for donating. Once approved by staff, egg donor profiles, along with current pictures, are posted on an agency's password-protected website under the woman's first name. The donor then waits to be selected by a recipient before undergoing medical, psychological, and genetic screening.

In contrast, sperm banks do not post profiles until donors pass the medical screening and produce enough samples to be listed for sale on the bank's publicly accessible website. Western Sperm Bank's donor manager explained,

> From the moment the donor is signed on, it's really nine months before we even see any profit from them. They have six months worth of quarantine [for HIV], and then another three months before we can really release enough inventory so that people aren't upset at us. If we release five vials and twenty women call, only two women are going to be happy. The others are going to be really upset that that's all we got on him this month.

Sperm banks are much more concerned about donor anonymity, so men's profiles are assigned an identification number and do not include current photographs.[7] Both banks do offer a "photo-matching service," in which recipients pay staff to select donors with specified phenotypes.

Profiles serve as the primary marketing tool for both the program and the donor. For donation programs, posted profiles represent the full range of donors available and thus are used to recruit recipient clients. The founder of Creative Beginnings explained that she would prefer not to have profiles on the website because she thinks they are impersonal but that she needs them to be "competitive" with other programs.[8] For donors, the profiles are the primary basis a recipient will use to select them. Typically, recipients also consult with staff about which donors to choose; occasionally, egg recipients will ask to meet a donor, but under no circumstances are sperm recipients allowed to meet donors. If a donor's profile is not appealing, recipients are not likely to express interest in purchasing that donor's sex cells.

This explains why programs spend a great deal of energy encouraging applicants to complete the profiles and, in the case of egg donation, to send in attractive pictures. During an informational meeting for women interested in becoming egg donors, Creative Beginnings' staff members offered explicit advice about how they should appeal to recipients.

ASSISTANT DIRECTOR: The profile really gives recipients a chance to get to know you on another level. Even though it's anonymous, it feels like it's personal. It feels like they're making a connection with you. They want to feel like it's less clinical than just looking it up on the website, and they want to see which girl best suits their needs. It's about who looks like they could fit into my family and who has the characteristics that I would like in my offspring? You can never be too conceited or too proud of your accomplishments because they really like to feel like, wow, this is a really special and unique person. And they want to feel like they're helping you just like you're helping them. They know that money is a good motivator, but they also want to feel like you're here for some altruistic purposes. So I always say to let your personality show, but also you can kind of look at the question and think, if I were in their position, how would I want somebody to answer that question? I don't want you to be somebody that you're not, but think of being sensitive to their needs and feelings when you're answering them. That's the big portion of it. The pictures are another portion. We always ask for one good head-and-shoulder shot. It's whatever is your best representation, flattering, and lets you come out.

DONOR ASSISTANT: You don't want something where your boobs are hanging out of your top [*laughter*]. These people are not looking for sexy people.

ASSISTANT DIRECTOR: We get girls who send in pictures from their homecoming dance, but everybody takes those pictures where they're half-wasted, and they've got their drink in one hand and their cigarette in another. Recipients don't need to see it. It's like your parents: ignorance is bliss.

Egg donors are encouraged by agency staff to construct properly feminine profiles for the recipients, who are continually referenced as an oblique "they" who will be reading the donors' answers and making judgments about their motivations. Although it is important for the "girls" to let their "personalities" shine through, the recipients do not necessarily need to know about their flaws, such as wearing revealing clothing, drinking, or smoking.[9]

If a donor's profile is deemed unacceptable by staff or if she sends in unattractive pictures, an agency will "delete" her from the database. Creative Beginnings' office manager explained, "We have to provide what our client wants, and that's a specific type of donor. Even though [the recipients] may not be the most beautiful people on the face of the earth, they want the best. So that's what we have to provide to them." In contrast, sperm recipients are not allowed to see photographs of donors, and thus men's physical appearance is not held to similarly high standards.

Sperm bank staff members will take extra time with men who discuss only financial motivations in their profiles, but they are much less explicit about the need to appear altruistic. This dynamic was made clear as Western Sperm Bank's donor manager explained how she came to understand the importance of profiles.

[Prior to this job,] when I worked on the infertility side, women [recipients] would come in with their little donor vials [of sperm]. Some of them would show me the [donor profile and say,] "Doesn't he sound wonderful?" And of course this is all they've got. This is their person, this little sheet. So [Western Sperm Bank's staff] will look at [the profile] and if someone's sort of negative will really question the donor. "Do you really mean that money is the only thing for you?" And if it is, we are honest enough to just leave it that way. But a lot of times [donors] say, "Well, it's not just the money, it's also. . . ." [So the staff will say,] "Why don't you rewrite this little portion to reflect that also?" The new [staff] became more conscious and willing to put in the effort to make more complete answers, because they did care about what was presented to the recipients, to give them a fuller image of what the person was like.

Although egg agencies specifically use the terms "help" and "altruism" in advising women who are writing their profiles, the sperm donor manager does not specify what other motivation the man is expected to have besides financial compensation. He is only supposed to revise his profile with the "also" in mind.

These gendered coaching strategies contribute to statistically significant differences in how women and men answer the profile question "Why do you want to be a donor?" Based on a content analysis of 826 donor profiles, Figure 2 reveals that the majority of egg donors at Ova-Corp, Creative Beginnings, and Gametes Inc. dutifully reported that they were interested in donation only because they wanted to help people. A small percentage of women reported being motivated both by altruism and financial considerations, but almost none said they were solely interested in the money. At the sperm banks, men are much less hesitant about stating their interest in the compensation, even though they are making much less money than women. And it is interesting to note that CryoCorp's profiles do not even include this question, in keeping with a general lack of interest in men's motivations.[10]

Although the distribution of profile responses among egg donors and among sperm donors is strikingly similar across programs, the reader is cautioned against seeing evidence of some "natural" difference between the sexes. As will be discussed more in Chapter 4, the majority of men *and*

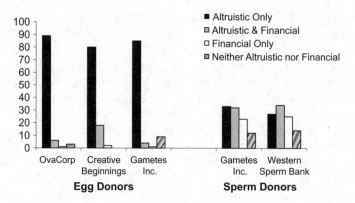

Figure 2. Percentage of women and men expressing altruistic and/or financial motivations on donor profiles, by program

women are drawn to donation by the financial incentives, but these initial interests are whittled into gender-appropriate responses on the donor profiles.

Both egg agencies and sperm banks believe that donor profiles offer recipient clients "reassurance". in the form of extensive information about the donor. The founder of Creative Beginnings explained that infertility "is emotionally devastating, and [recipients] feel like they have no control. So those first appointments, sometimes people are really excited about the profiles, because they want to see what the people are like that we are going to be supplying to them. They're really happy when they see the quality of the donor and the amount of information they get." Similarly, the donor screener at Western Sperm Bank noted that "it's hard on the recipient end to be taking this leap of faith, buying reproductive fluid from unseen, unknown strangers, so I understand the desire to know as much as you possibly can. So we try to glean stories about [the donors], and then it's just nice reassurance for the recipients that these are real people." In the same breath, staff members draw on both economic and social understandings to describe donors as "real people" who are "supplied" to recipients.

Egg agencies and sperm banks use donor profiles to recruit clients, and recipients who select particular women and men based on details about eye color, family health history, favorite movie, and SAT scores begin to think of the donor as that profile. But donors are not producing unmediated texts that travel from keyboard to website display. Gendered cultural norms, formalized through organizational processes, result in expectations that women reflect altruistic sentiments beneath an attractive photograph, and sperm donors are vaguely encouraged to provide a "fuller image." Although the recipient is actually buying eggs or sperm, these sex cells become personified through the donor profile, and it is this gendered, commodified personification of the donor that the recipient is purchasing.

MATCHMAKING

When a recipient chooses a specific donor, it is called a "match." In egg agencies, the selected donor will then be medically and psychologically screened before she signs a legal contract with "her couple." In sperm banks, there is a limited "inventory" of vials from each donor, and this supply is replenished as men continue to make regular deposits throughout their yearlong commitment to the bank.[11] The vials are listed in the bank's "catalog," so a recipient who calls to place an order is advised to choose two or three different sperm donors to ensure that at least one will be available for purchase.

Matches are the primary source of income for agencies and banks, and the staff works hard to confirm them. Recipients are urged to browse donor profiles, but staff members will also take the time to discuss various donors' attributes, thereby shaping recipients' perceptions. This intermediary role is made clear in the following excerpt, which is one side of a telephone conversation between Creative Beginnings' founder and a recipient who is in the process of choosing a donor.

FOUNDER: We have a donor that I'd like you to look at. . . .

She just donated in the last couple of days, 27 eggs, and she had 23 beautiful embryos. And her name is Meredith. . . .

She is beautiful and bright and tall, and she has a degree in fine arts, I think, and she's a student, a real good student. . . .

Photography school . . .

It's a good place for us to get donors [*laughs*]. All that equipment and film costs a lot of money. . . .

She's a really bright, classy lady. . . .

Take a look at Meredith; she's a great opportunity. . . .

And I think Heidi would be a great choice. . . .

I love 'em all! . . .

And check out Heidi, too, because she's still an option for you but not much longer. People are going to go after her soon. Somebody's going to grab Meredith, too, because she just finished a cycle. . . .

No, it would be like six weeks before she could do one. . . .

But Heidi is ready to go. . . .

Go look. . . .

Okay, bye; you're welcome.

Both the donor and her embryos are labeled "beautiful," and she is "bright" and "a really good student," which provides an innocuous explanation for why she needs money from egg donation. Positive descriptions such as these help agencies create a sense of urgency about the donor being "grabbed" by some other recipient if the caller does not act quickly. These sorts of pressure tactics are helpful in confirming a match because as OvaCorp's donor manager explained, "99.9% of the time [recipients] will go with a donor], especially if they know someone else is waiting."

Although recipients learn details about donors from the profiles and staff, this flow of information does not go both ways. Sperm donors at CryoCorp and Western Sperm Bank are not given any information about who purchases their sperm. Creative Beginnings' egg donors are often given vague, nonidentifying information (e.g., the recipients are "schoolteachers in their forties who have been trying for a long time to have children"). OvaCorp's egg donors are given a short letter written by the recipients explaining why they are using egg donation. Program mangers see this information as quite motivating for egg donors. OvaCorp's psychologist called it an "obvious rule of thumb about human nature," encouraging recipients to "Please call [the donor], stay in touch. She'll do a better job for you if she knows you care." The founder of the second major egg agency on the West Coast agreed, stating,

> I believe that a donor has a right to [an] important, honest, nonidentifiable evaluation of the recipient. That's how they let go. To say "You're going to give an egg and you'll never know anything about it and we're going to give you $5,000," it's a business transaction. Versus "We're going to give you $5,000, thank you for what you're going through, you're answering someone's prayer, and you're changing their lives. They have two Dalmatians. He's a fireman. She's always dreamed of being a mother. She's had two miscarriages. Their lives have stopped. You're changing them. They're going to raise this child with so much love." There's a real big difference for the donor.

Egg agencies find some donors easier to match than others. The most sought-after are "repeat donors," who have proven their reliability by completing at least one donation cycle, or "proven donors," whose eggs have resulted in pregnancy for a previous recipient, thus providing evidence of fertility. All sperm donors are screened for exceptionally high sperm counts, so banks do not label their donors as "proven." In fact, neither sperm bank had ever considered dropping a donor whose sperm had not resulted in any pregnancies. Some donors are also labeled "popular" because their profiles generate almost daily calls from potential recipients visiting the website. OvaCorp's donor manager, leafing through a profile she had just received, said, "I can tell when I can match a girl quick."

> Well number one, she's attractive. Number two, she has a child, which is a huge plus. I mean look [*shows Rene her picture and profile*]. And the kindest woman. She has a really good background. See, definitely it's not for the money. She makes 65 grand a year. Great height and weight. Obviously Hispanic, and I start reading a little bit about her, and she has phenomenal answers about why she wants to do this. She's given the couple total leadership, and that's wonderful. She can travel because she's in Texas. So she'd be an easy match. Young, twenty-six, young child. There's definitely proven fertility. 5 feet 7 inches, 110 [pounds]. She's Caucasian

enough. She's white enough to pass, but she has a nice good hue to her if you have a Hispanic couple. Educated, good family health history. Very outgoing. Easy match. Easy match.

This stream-of-consciousness perusal of a donor profile reveals the intersection of sex and gender with race and class in defining popular donors. The donor's own child attests to her body's ability to create pregnancy-producing eggs. Her relatively high salary and eloquence on the page demonstrate her altruism. And her "hue" makes her phenotypically flexible to match either Caucasian or Hispanic recipients.

FEES

One of the most striking comparisons in this market is how egg agencies and sperm banks pay women and men for sex cells. The most obvious difference is the level of compensation; per donation, egg donors are generally paid around $5,000, and sperm donors are paid around $75. Of course, there are enormous differences in what is required of women to produce eggs and men to produce sperm (discussed in more detail in Chapter 3), particularly in terms of physical risk, a rationale for the difference in fees that is referenced both by the ASRM's Ethics Committee and program staff.[12] In the succinct words of one physician–researcher: "The egg donor goes through a lot more, and they're paid more."

However, when one compares the rate per contract, the difference is not so extreme; it takes women a month or two to complete a cycle, and men agree to donate at least once a week for a year. By the end of the year, men's total earnings may begin to approach women's, but women can complete several donations in that time as long as they continue to attract recipient interest. Moreover, women's fees generally increase with each cycle, especially if a previous donation resulted in pregnancy, so an egg donor's annual earnings can quickly outpace a sperm donor's.

Because of biological sex differences, it is difficult to justify a direct comparison of the *amount* paid to women and men, but it is possible to compare other aspects of how programs manage the financial compensation. First, women who complete a cycle are paid regardless of how many eggs they produce, yet men are paid only if the sample meets bank standards for sperm count. Otherwise, men receive nothing for that day's donation, a form of piecework compensation in which payment is based on production. Second, egg agencies pay women in one lump sum, usually after the retrieval surgery.[13] Men are paid every two weeks, mimicking the schedule and format of a paycheck that one would receive as an employee in a workplace. Third, sperm banks pay the same flat rate to each of their donors, but egg agencies often adjust a donor's compensation based on her personal characteristics.

Indeed, the final stage of confirming an egg donor match is negotiating the donor's fee, which can be affected by her performance in previous cycles, her education level, and even her race/ethnicity. During an interview in 2002, an OvaCorp staffer explained how "the donors range."

> They start at $3,500, but if you're Asian, you command a higher fee. If you're highly educated, there's no set number. If you have a degree, you'll get more than if you're a high school graduate. If you're a successful repeater, [that is,] couples have had a child by you, then you're a better bet than to go through the cycle with a newcomer and nothing happens, or she produces two eggs. A successful repeater could get $12,000 for her eggs. We have a few that are just exceptional, where everyone's gotten pregnant, they're brilliant, they're beautiful, they're educated.

Due to the difficulty of maintaining a diverse pool of donors, both egg agencies often increase the fee for donors of color, especially Asian Americans and African Americans. This results in a situation where they are often more highly valued than white women, which is unexpected, given that the reverse is often true in other contexts, including the labor market and in adoption agencies. But in this market, race is seen as a biologically based characteristic, and sex cells from women of color are perceived as scarce, which contributes to their increased value.

In determining appropriate fees for particular donors, egg agency staffers often consult with one another. In this excerpt from a weekly staff meeting at OvaCorp, the donor manager and her assistant discuss with the agency director a match between a wealthy recipient and a donor they call "an ace in the hole" and a "sure bet," because her eggs consistently result in recipient pregnancies.

DONOR MANAGER: We're going with Helen. I told her she was getting 10 [thousand dollars].

DONOR ASSISTANT: [The recipient] said, "I don't care what she's asking for." He says, "I want a baby."

DIRECTOR: I always felt that we would give her maybe 12 [thousand dollars]. She's done it so many times.

DONOR MANAGER: Well, why don't we give her 12 [thousand dollars] on confirmation of pregnancy?

DIRECTOR: Yeah, something like that. Just because she's gone so many times.

DONOR MANAGER: She's made a whole bunch of money.

DIRECTOR: And the [recipients] can afford it.

DONOR MANAGER: So why don't we do it as a gift?

DIRECTOR: Yeah. We'll do 10 [thousand dollars] and then 2,000 [dollars] on confirmation of pregnancy or first trimester or whatever you want to do. You know there's going to be a pregnancy.

In addition to reflecting the widespread use of gift rhetoric in egg agencies, this discussion also highlights the continuing intermediary role played by staffers, as they determine what recipients can afford while also securing the highest possible fee for women, in part to cultivate donor loyalty in a metropolitan area with several other egg agencies. If recipients are perceived as wealthy, the staff members will often ask for a higher donor fee, as when a program assistant at one egg agency mentioned that "gay men, single men have a lot of money, and they think nothing of 7, 8 thousand dollars." However, staffers do not appreciate it when requests for higher fees come from the donors. Creative Beginnings' founder expressed "disappointment" in "girls that really ask you to negotiate," saying, "I really don't like that. It's really uncomfortable, and couples don't like it."[14]

There are literally hundreds of other donors available, either within a given program or at nearby programs, so it appears that these fees are not as responsive to supply and demand as one would expect. Unfortunately, there are no aggregate statistics available to measure "supply" (number of donors or number of gametes produced) or "demand" (number of recipients or quantity of gametes consumed), which makes it difficult to test this claim rigorously. However, it has been noted by other observers of this market.[15] There is also a dearth of data about the financial situations of egg and sperm recipients, which leaves open questions about the extent to which they are able to afford assisted reproduction. Such calculations would be further complicated by a patchwork of state mandates and insurance policies, some of which provide coverage for donor insemination or IVF.

In an attempt to capture the supply of sex cells available at the egg agencies and sperm banks in this study, Figure 3 illustrates the number of donors with profiles posted in each program.[16] At the egg agencies, the white part of the bar reflects the number of egg donors who are currently matched to recipients, which renders them unavailable to other recipients and thus provides some evidence of demand. OvaCorp, one of the largest and oldest egg agencies in the country, cataloged 465 donors and had 100 active donor/recipient matches in the summer of 2002. That same summer, Creative Beginnings, a new egg agency that had been open for just three years, already had 123 egg donors listed online, with 23 women in active matches. In 2006, Gametes Inc., a sperm bank that had been open for thirty years, posted just 113 sperm donors, and its egg agency, which had opened just a few years before, already had profiles for 75 women, 25 of whom were matched. In 2002, CryoCorp, one of the largest and oldest sperm banks in the country, listed 125 donors, and Western Sperm Bank, the small, nonprofit program, had vials from just 30 donors. In terms of recipient demand for men's gametes, CryoCorp reports distributing about 2,500 vials every month, and Western Sperm Bank estimates that it serves around 400 recipients each year.[17]

It is certainly the case that egg agencies and sperm banks have different business models. Egg agencies are essentially brokers, matching donors and recipients before sending them off to medical professionals for tests and procedures. In 2002, both OvaCorp and Creative Beginnings

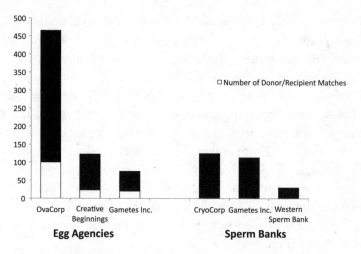

Figure 3. Number of egg and sperm donors with posted profiles, by program

charged recipients an agency fee of $3,500 for these services and then added standard fees for the donor's medical and legal expenses. The egg donor's fee is a separate line item on the bill, and the agency receives no additional compensation for negotiating a higher fee for her. If recipients experience a "failed cycle" with a donor, the staff might offer a discounted rate on the second cycle. In some cases, staff will even explain the situation to the egg donor and ask her to accept a lower fee.

Sperm banks are much more than brokerages in that they have labs for testing sperm samples, storage facilities for freezing thousands of vials in nitrogen tanks, and shipping departments for managing distribution. In 2002, the nonprofit Western Sperm Bank paid men $50 for each acceptable sample, and the for-profit CryoCorp paid $75. Acceptable samples can generally be split into several vials, from two or three to as many as eight or nine. Each vial is then sold for $175 at Western Sperm Bank and $215 at CryoCorp.[18] Undoubtedly, the different business models contribute to the different prices in this market.

Another consideration for an analysis of supply and demand is the unexpected finding that sperm donors are relatively difficult to recruit, yet egg donors sign up en masse. With very little advertising, OvaCorp receives around one hundred applications a day, and Creative Beginnings receives several hundred inquiries every month. In stark contrast, CryoCorp maintains three locations in different parts of the country and employs several people whose entire job description revolves around donor recruitment. Moreover, both sperm banks pay current donors hundreds of dollars in "finder's fees" if they refer applicants who are accepted into the program. Discussing his experience running a sperm bank, the founder of Gametes Inc. explained,

> For a substantial part of our history, donor recruitment was a major concern, having an aggregate number of donors plus donor diversity. We just couldn't keep inventory to meet the demand. Not that we were growing hugely. You'd think if you didn't have enough inventory to meet demand, then you could name your own price and just be fabulously wealthy. Well, it didn't work out that way.

To increase the supply of sperm, Gametes Inc. opened offices around their small Southern town. In doing so, according to the founder, they were "taking a page from financial bankers who have branches on every corner. You'd think convenience would be a major asset. Well, most guys don't want people knowing that they're masturbating, so having a neighborhood branch where mom and dad can see what you're doing isn't really cool [laughs]." Over the years, the program opened offices in a nearby university town, in a large city a few hours away, in a nearby state, and in Canada. But now, it maintains just two offices: "headquarters" in the same small Southern city where the program started and a satellite office in a large city two hours away that is close to several major universities. To this day, Gametes Inc. must advertise constantly for sperm donors, and program staffers routinely remind men to send in their friends.

It is striking that the difficulty in recruiting men does not produce an increase in their compensation and the apparent oversupply of women has not caused their fees to drop. Two popular conceptions—that most men would jump at the chance to make some extra cash by selling their sperm and that it is difficult to find women willing to undergo shots and surgery for $5,000—simply do not hold. Indeed, between 2002 and 2008, the number of profiles listed on OvaCorp's website more than doubled.

The program now has more than a thousand women available to donate, yet recipients are still informed that egg donor fees will be between $5,000 and $10,000.

In this stage of the process, a donor's attributes, encapsulated in the profile and extolled by staff, are used to generate income for the programs through matches, but the economic valuation of women's eggs is more intimate than that of men's sperm. Women are paid to produce eggs for a particular recipient who has agreed to a specific price for that donor's sex cells. At the same time, staffers tell recipients the "donor would love to work with you," and they inform egg donors that the recipients just "loved you and had to have you." Thus, egg agencies structure the exchange not only as a legalistic economic transaction, but also as the beginning of a caring gift cycle, which the staff members foster by expressing appreciation to the egg donors, both on behalf of the agency and the agency's clients.

OvaCorp's donor manager explained, "We have the largest donor database. The reason is we treat them like royalty. They are women, not genetics, to us. A lot of times a couple doesn't meet them, so we want them to feel our warmth, feel the reality that we're so grateful for what they're doing for us as well as because they're making our couple happy." Likewise, CryoCorp's marketing director notes, "We have to walk that tightrope and make sure the [sperm] donors are happy, because if we don't have happy donors, then we don't have a program, and yet make sure the clients are happy as well [laughs]. So we're always mindful of that." But in sperm banks, being a "happy donor," whose sex cells are purchased by many different recipients months after he has produced them, is not predicated on being placed in the position of "loving" and "being loved by" extremely grateful "future parents."

FRAMING PAID DONATION AS A GIFT OR A JOB

Programs screen applicants for "responsibility," and staff must carefully monitor donors as they fulfill contractual obligations to produce eggs and sperm. Egg agency staffers are always on the phone with donors and doctors to find out when women begin menstruating, start fertility shots, miss doctors' appointments, and schedule egg retrievals. Creative Beginnings' founder explained, "Most of the donors are very conscientious, and especially our donors, because we look for girls who are going to be compliant and do things right." To maintain "inventory," sperm bank staffers are continually assessing which donors miss appointments, register unusually low sperm counts, or need blood drawn for periodic disease testing. According to a donor screener, Western Sperm Bank must be vigilant because donors "are creating a product that we're vouching for in terms of quality control."

If an egg donor is not currently available, as is the case with many of the most popular donors, then an egg recipient can "reserve" her for a future cycle. If a sperm donor's vials are "sold out" for that month, recipients can be placed on a waiting list. Sperm recipients also have the option of creating a "storage account," in which they buy multiple vials of a particular donor's sperm to guarantee its availability if they do not become pregnant during initial inseminations. In explaining this system, CryoCorp's marketing director blurs the line between the donor and the donor's sperm when she discussed the bank's "inventory."

> We do limit the number of vials available on any given donor by limiting the amount of time a donor can be in the program. All of our specimens are available on a first-come, first-serve basis. We are dealing with human beings here, and the donors have finals and they don't come in. And they go away for the summer. So our inventory is somewhat variable. So we suggest [recipients] open a storage account, which just costs a little bit additionally, and then purchase as many vials as they want.

In each of the four programs, staffers identify the donor's responsibilities as being like those in a job, but in the case of egg donation, it is understood to be much more meaningful than any regular job. At an informational meeting for potential egg donors, Creative Beginnings' founder explained, "You get paid really well, and so you have to do all the things you do for a normal job. You have to show up at the right time and place and do what's expected of you." Her assistant added, "If you really simplify the math, it's $4,000 for six weeks of work, and it's maybe a couple hours a day, if that. And to know that you're doing something positive and amazing in somebody's life and then getting compensated for it, you can't ask for anything better than that." Agency staffers simultaneously tell potential egg donors to think of donation "like a job" while also embedding the women's responsibility in the "amazing" task of helping others.

Contact between staff and donors does not necessarily end on the day of the egg retrieval or when sperm donors provide their last sample. Sperm donors must return to the bank for HIV testing six months after they stop donating, and men who agree to release identifying information to offspring must update their addresses with the bank indefinitely. If an egg donor performs well in her first cycle, then the agency will hope to match her with future recipients. However, OvaCorp's donor manager is careful not to ask a woman too early about another cycle. She explained, "If it's a first-timer, I won't ask her to do it again until she's cleared the cycle, because I don't want her to think I'm being insistent upon a mass producer. I'll say, 'There's another couple that would love to work with you. However, let's just concentrate on this one couple that we're talking about.'"

But women who attempt to make a "career" of selling eggs provoke disgust among staff, in part because they violate the altruistic framing of donation. Egg agencies generally follow ASRM guidelines limiting women to five cycles, recommendations that are designed to minimize health risks. However, it is not concern for the woman's health that the OvaCorp donor manager expresses in this denunciation of one such "career" egg donor. "She's done this as a professional. It's like a career now. I said, 'There's something about that girl.' Then I called [the director of another egg agency], and she's like 'oh yeah, why's she calling you? I won't work with her anymore; she worked with me eight times.' I said, 'Eight times?! She's got four kids. She's on the county. Yeah, I remember that name.'"

In sperm banks, the decision to limit men's donations centers on the goal of efficiently running a business without offending the sensibilities of the bank's clients. CryoCorp's CEO explained,

> There's an ongoing debate of how many vials should you collect from any one donor. If you have 10 donors and collect 10,000 vials from all of them and you have to replace 1 [donor because of genetic or medical is-

sues], it's taking a hit to your business. If you wind up with 10,000 donors and only collect 10 vials from every single one, you're inefficiently operating your business. You need to figure out what that sweet spot is. But then there's the emotional issue from a purchaser. If a client knows that, with X thousand vials out there, there could be 100 or 200 offspring, what's that point where it just becomes emotionally too many? With my MBA hat on, we are not collecting enough vials per donor, because we're not operating as efficiently as we should. With my customer relations/consumer hat on, we're collecting the right number of vials, because clients perceive that it's important to keep that number to something emotionally tolerable. At what point do you say that's just not someone I want to be the so-called father of my child, because there's just way too many possible brothers and sisters out there?

Given the extensive investment required to screen gamete donors, one would expect programs to gather as much reproductive material as possible from each person. Instead, women are discouraged from becoming "professional" egg donors, and men are prevented from "fathering" too many offspring.

In keeping with the focus on altruism in egg donation, both OvaCorp and Creative Beginnings' staffers encourage recipients to send the donor a thank-you note after the egg retrieval. This behavior is not present in the sperm banks. In many cases, egg recipients also give the donor flowers, jewelry, or an additional financial gift, thereby upholding the constructed vision of egg donation as reciprocal gift giving, in which donors help recipients and recipients help donors. Creative Beginnings' founder explained that if recipients ask her "about getting flowers for the donors, I ask them not to do that, because flowers get in the way. The donor's sleeping, and she's not thinking about flowers. If you want to get a gift, get a simple piece of jewelry, because then the donor has something forever that she did something really nice." This rhetoric even shapes accounting practices; although most programs inform donors that they will be sent a 1099 tax form, which is designed for independent contractors providing a service, one of the egg agencies considers the donor's fee a nontaxable "gift" from the recipient.

The most extreme case I heard of postcycle giving was reported by OvaCorp's donor manager.

Donor Manager: I paid a donor $25,000. That's only because it was $10,000 for the donor's fee, and then when their kids were born, they gave her an additional gift of $15,000.

Rene: Are you serious?
Donor Manager: Oh yeah. That was a gift to her. They said, "What do we do?" Well, you bought me and [the donor] a pair of $3,000 earrings. They're a very wealthy couple. I love them. She had [the earrings] made by somebody in Italy. Mine had rubies at the end of them, the donor's had emeralds, and the couple's, hers had sapphires. So when her girls were born, she says "Maybe I'll get her some more earrings." I said "The likelihood of her wearing those earrings is very slim [because] she's really low key." I said "Give her a financial compensation." She's like, "Okay, I'll give her $15,000, 7,500 [dollars] per girl." She had twins.

Here, the monetary value of the recipient's gift to the donor is explicitly tied to the number of children she had as a result of the donor's eggs, making the line between gift and sale indistinguishable.

In egg donation, the earlier stage of fee negotiation gives way to an understanding that donors are providing a gift to which recipients are expected to respond with a thank-you note, and many choose to give the donor a gift of their own. In sperm donation, men are far more likely to be treated like employees, clocking in at the sperm bank at least once a week to produce a "high-quality" sample. Indeed, this framing of donation as a job leads some men to be so removed from what they are donating that when a new employee at Western Sperm Bank excitedly told a donor that a recipient had become pregnant with his samples, she said it was like "somebody hit him with this huge ball in the middle of his head. He just went blank, and he was shocked." During his next visit, the sperm donor explained, "I hadn't really thought about the fact there were gonna be pregnancies." The donor manager described this state of mind as "not uncommon."

Anthropologist Rayna Rapp observes that "Contemporary biomedical rationality . . . [is] operating to reproduce older forms of gender, ethnoracial, class, and national stratification even (or perhaps especially) on its technologically 'revolutionary' edges."[19] Indeed, these portrayals of altruistic femininity and emotionally distant masculinity fit a very traditional pattern, and the sperm donor's reaction exposes the reflexive application of gendered norms in this medical market. Although most egg donors will never meet their genetic children, they are still expected to be "naturally" caring, guiltily hiding any interest they might have in the promise of thousands of dollars. This is a form of emotional work not required of men donating sperm, even though they are more likely to be contacted by their biological offspring through the banks' identity-release programs.

ONE PROGRAM, TWO KINDS OF DONATION

Donor insemination and *in vitro* fertilization developed at different times in distinct spheres of scientific research. Many early commercial programs were started by people with links to these worlds, so they generally offered egg donation or sperm donation but not both. This division of the market into sex-specific firms continues to the present, with most programs specializing in one or the other. To assess whether the gendered protocols that exist at CryoCorp, Western Sperm Bank, Creative Beginnings, and OvaCorp persist even in organizations that sell both eggs and sperm, I turn briefly to daily business practices at Gametes Inc. and University Fertility Services.

Gametes Inc. was one of the first commercial sperm banks to open in the United States, but it was nearly thirty years before it decided to get into the egg donation business. The founder of Gametes Inc. derided other egg agencies as simply offering "picture galleries" of attractive young women, and he decided his company would medically and psychologically screen prospective donors *before* posting their profiles to its website. He hired new staff members, and within just three years, Gametes Inc. had compiled a roster of 75 women who were willing to donate their eggs, a surprising figure given that the sperm bank offered samples from just 112 men after so many years of being open.

In starting the egg agency, though, Gametes Inc. did not follow the model it had established at its sperm bank. The new staffers hired to run the egg agency worked in a different wing of the building, and they were sometimes surprised when I pointed out the differences in protocols that each program had developed. For example, the sperm bank had an elaborate identity-release program, one in which it paid men 50% more per sample if they consented to release identifying information to offspring. In contrast, the egg agency, like most egg agencies, had no such program and even refused to give egg donors basic information about whether their recipients had become pregnant or not, a direct contrast to the more open egg agencies on the West Coast. Examples such as this underscore the extent to which there is gendered bifurcation in program protocols. However, the fact that the content of those protocols can be so variable provides further evidence that there is nothing inherent in biology or technology that determines particular policies.

There is also evidence of the gendered framing of egg and sperm donation at Gametes Inc. Gametes Inc.'s egg agency created its own distinct website, which differed in both design and organization from the sperm bank's website, and each program asked prospective donors to fill out gender-specific applications with different questions for women and men. Staffers joked around with sperm donors, offering them free T-shirts and key chains with funny slogans, but egg agency staffers thanked women for their gift with Fabergé-esque eggs or small hearts at the end of a cycle. One similarity between the egg and sperm branches of Gametes Inc. is that both offer adult photos of donors; its sperm bank is one of the few in the country to do so. However, just 27% of men's profiles included adult photos, compared to 92% of women's profiles.

At University Fertility Services, there had been an active sperm donation program for years when nurse–coordinators began recruiting egg donors. In organizing both kinds of donation, staff members offered recipients very little information about donors, and they maintained strict anonymity, as at other university programs on the East Coast. The similarity ends there, though. As at Gametes Inc., there were different screening protocols for and expectations of women and men. For example, during a period in the 1990s, the same person was responsible for screening both egg and sperm donors, and she used the same preliminary questionnaire. However, many of the egg donors' forms included a scribbled note about why the woman was interested in being a donor (e.g., "why—wants to help" or "why—loves kids"). Not a single one of the sperm donors' forms includes these handwritten notations about motivations.[20] By the time I conducted research there in 2006, the sperm donor program was no longer active, but this question about women's motivations had been formally incorporated into the intake questionnaire for egg donor applicants.

The different expectations of egg and sperm donors are made especially clear in this discussion with a prominent physician–researcher who had served as medical director of University Fertility Services for two decades. When asked how he would define a great egg donor, in addition to discussing her medical and reproductive history, he explained,

Physician: I like to see some altruism of the [egg] donors. Yes, we pay them $2,000, and that's probably the low end of what donors are getting paid around the nation, but in [this small college town], it's not an insignificant amount of money. When we ask them, "Why do you want to be a donor?" most say, "Well, I saw this [news] program on TV, or I've got a cousin that's going through infertility, or I want to help people." Most of them, it's about some reason other than I saw an ad in the newspaper, and I want to make some money, because it's a hard way of making money.

Rene: What is it about altruism that's important?
Physician: It just tells me that they're less likely to have regrets down the road, that they've really approached this as "I want to help somebody," not "I'm doing this to make money."

Rene: And then a similar question for sperm donors. What would make you think this is a great donor?
Physician: The sperm donors were different. They weren't paid very much per specimen. I think it was 50 bucks. Sperm donors, in general, weren't as altruistic. They honestly were guys that wanted to make money, and guys have less attachment of their sperm than women do of their eggs. Very few sperm donors actually ever have regrets about, you know, "What did I do?" So, men were a little different than the women.

In summarizing attitudes toward the men and women who provide sex cells for infertility patients, a lab technician who had worked at University Fertility Services since the late 1980s said, "I think a lot of people felt that sperm donors were a dime a dozen and your egg donors are gold."

CONCLUSION

Casual observers of the medical market for sex cells point to biological differences between women and men and consider them explanation enough for the greater economic and cultural valuation of egg donors. Indeed, individual women have fewer eggs than individual men have sperm, and egg retrieval requires surgery, while sperm retrieval requires masturbation. However, shifting the lens from individual bodies to the broader market reveals an oversupply of women willing to be egg donors. Both the yearlong commitment and stringent requirements make men difficult to recruit, yet hundreds of women's profiles languish on agency websites, far outstripping recipient demand. Despite this abundance, egg donor fees hold steady and are often calibrated by staff perceptions of a woman's characteristics and a recipient's wealth. Moreover, these high levels of compensation coexist seamlessly with altruistic rhetoric, because agency staff members draw on cultural norms of maternal femininity to frame egg donation as a gift exchange.

It is not that altruistic rhetoric is completely absent in sperm banks or that men cannot make a couple of thousand dollars a year providing weekly samples, but the dynamic interplay between biological, economic, cultural, and structural factors differentiates the market for eggs from that for sperm in each stage of the donation process. In recruiting marketable donors, both egg agencies and sperm banks place advertisements listing biological requirements (e.g., age), but egg agencies emphasize the opportunity to help and sperm banks portray donation as a job, a distinction shaped by gendered stereotypes that appear in countless organizational processes. The greater cultural acceptance of egg donation probably results in more women applicants than men, and staffers screen women based on biological factors such as medical history. But also under review are a woman's physical appearance and stated motivations. Men's health history is similarly scrutinized, and those willing to release identifying information to offspring are preferred, but responsibility, height, and sperm count ultimately define the ideal sperm donor.

Once accepted into a donation program, a woman's profile will be used to match her with a specific recipient client, as eggs cannot yet be frozen like sperm.[21] Men must build enough "inventory" for their profiles to be posted to the program's website, and their vials are available on a first-come, first-serve basis. Stored by the hundreds in large tanks, men's donations resemble a standardized product more so than the eggs that are removed from an individual woman and placed into "her" recipient a few days later. This is probably partly responsible for the different approaches to compensation, in which men are paid a set rate only for those samples deemed acceptable. Although most egg donors receive the market rate, it is common for a woman's characteristics (such as prior donations, education level, and race) to increase her fee. The personal, one-to-one relationship between altruistic egg donor and grateful egg recipient is codified into an actual gift exchange when staff members encourage recipients to write a thank-you letter or provide a small token of appreciation. Bank staffers do not request similar displays of gratitude for sperm donors.

Neither biological differences between women and men nor economic laws of supply and demand fully explain the medical market for sex cells. Reproductive cells and reproductive bodies are filtered through economic and cultural lenses in a particular organizational context—that of medicalized egg agencies and sperm banks. It is not just that individual women have fewer eggs than individual men have sperm, or that eggs are more difficult to extract, that produces both high prices and constant gift-talk in egg donation, but the close connection between women's reproductive bodies and cultural norms of caring motherhood. In contrast, men are much more difficult to recruit, yet they are paid low, standardized prices, and sperm donation is seen as more job than gift. As a result, both eggs and egg donors are more highly valued than sperm and sperm donors in this medical marketplace, where it is not just reproductive material but visions of maternal femininity and paternal masculinity that are marketed and purchased.

PART TWO Experiencing the Market

THREE Producing Eggs and Sperm

In the medical market for eggs and sperm, women and men are paid money to produce sex cells, a practice referred to as "donation" by egg agencies and sperm banks alike. However, egg donation is organized as a gift exchange, while sperm donation is likened to paid employment. In the second part of the book, I turn from the staff to the donors and ask whether these gendered framings of donation affect women's and men's experiences of bodily commodification. In each of the next three chapters, I approach this question from a different angle. First, I examine how egg and sperm donors experience the physical processes of donation; then, I compare how they think about the money they receive; and finally, I analyze how they respond to the possibility of children being born from their donations.

In this chapter, I focus on egg and sperm donors' embodied experiences, paying particular attention to how those experiences are shaped by the social context of paid donation. Most of what we know about the physical experience of *in vitro* fertilization is based on studies of infertile women, who turn to the technology in hopes of conceiving a child. In going through the first part of an IVF cycle, egg donors encounter the same regimen as infertile women: they inject the same medications, attend the same monitoring appointments, and endure the same egg retrieval surgery.[1] Because they are subject to the same technological processes, one might expect that infertile women and egg donors would have very similar physical reactions to the shots and surgery. However, the social context in which these two groups of women experience IVF is very different. Infertile women usually spend tens of thousands of dollars and months, if not years, of their lives trying to become pregnant. Egg donors are young, healthy women who receive thousands of dollars to give the gift of life. This raises the question of whether being paid to undergo IVF affects women's physical experiences of the technology.

In contrast, sperm donation does not require participation in risk-bearing medical procedures. Men must simply masturbate on a regular basis in the sperm bank, alternating their deposits with periods of abstinence. Scholars know little about men's experiences of masturbation, so it is an open question whether these are affected by variation in social context, that is in doing it for fun in one's bedroom versus doing it for money in the sperm bank. In detailing their activities, egg and sperm donors offer insight into the embodied experience of donating sex cells for money and provide evidence that the social context in which physical experiences occur can produce variation in how the body feels.

THE EMBODIED EXPERIENCE OF EGG DONATION

Research on the experiences of infertile women who are using IVF to conceive children suggests that it can be extremely disruptive to lives, careers, and marriages. The technology is portrayed as "all-consuming," and infertile women routinely describe feeling like they are on an "emotional roller coaster." In Sarah Franklin's study, many of the infertile women quit their jobs so as to manage the physical and emotional consequences of the treatment. She writes, "Women [repeatedly] emphasized that they did not realize how demanding the technique would be, how intensely it would affect them, and how much their lives would feel as though they had been 'taken over.'" Here are descriptions from two of Franklin's respondents.

> Jeanette Ives: It's a very intense procedure and if you're up at the hospital every day virtually and you are being monitored all the time so obviously it's a very intense time and you do get very involved in it all. Much more so than you imagine you will do, it's not like having one injection, you know, it's really involved. . . . And it does sort of take over your life to quite a big extent.

> Mary Chadwick: I didn't know what hit me, I honestly didn't know what hit me, I couldn't believe the intensity of the programme. . . . All you do is eat, drink, and talk IVF, your dinner conversation revolves around how big your follicles were that day, which side you had your injection in and that sort of thing, you just do, you just live and die IVF.[2]

In another interview study, Gay Becker finds that as women become immersed in biomedical fixes for infertility, they may experience "depersonalization" and begin to view their bodies as "defective."[3]

The question is whether egg donors offer similar accounts or whether being paid to undergo these procedures and not hoping for a long-awaited pregnancy alters the physical experiences of IVF. In fact, in explaining how the shots and surgery fit into their daily lives, egg donors described a very different embodied experience of the technology. They use matter-of-fact language to report each step required, from learning how to inject medications to attending medical appointments and recovering from egg retrieval surgery.

Shots and Surgery

The nineteen egg donors I interviewed had participated in a total of 42.5 cycles, including those in progress at the time we spoke.[4] Most of the women had cycled once or twice, but their experiences varied. Two donors had been matched with recipients but not yet donated, and one woman had already completed six cycles and was matched for a seventh. Two of the women had donated years before, but in most cases, the donation experience was much more recent; six women were in the midst of cycles, and five had cycled within the last two months.[5] Almost half the egg donors had a future cycle to which they were committed. In addition to participating in cycles organized by OvaCorp, Creative Beginnings, Gametes Inc., and University Fertility Services, some women had donated through other commercial agencies and university programs, and one had donated to a close friend. Within each program, women are sent to a variety of physicians, depending on where the recipient is receiving treatment. Thus, those who had signed on with multiple programs or cycled multiple times could compare their experiences with different programs and different physicians. (More details about the interviews and the donors are available in the Introduction and appendixes.)

Most of the egg donors had no previous experience with giving themselves shots, so the first step was to learn how to mix and inject the fertility medications. Heather, a senior in college, described how the nurse coordinator at University Fertility Services "showed me how to use the needles. The hormones and all the medicine come in one bottle, and then you have to syringe it out. She had to teach me how to flick all the bubbles out of the needle, how to clean the area, and make sure everything is sanitary."

Those bubbles worried Megan, another college student, who called the founder of Creative Beginnings before her first shot, concerned that she "couldn't get all the itty bitty microscopic bubbles. [The founder] said, 'It's okay; it's not going into your vein. It's going intramuscularly, so you won't have to worry. You won't get a blood clot in your brain, and you won't die [laughs].' I said, 'Okay, just curious [laughs].' Because it was a Saturday or Sunday and the doctors weren't there." Several donors indicated that they were nervous about giving themselves a shot the first time, and many turned to roommates or family members for help with the injection.

Like Megan, most egg donors described the staff at egg agencies and medical practices as readily available to answer questions. Rosa could call her nurse at "any time, midnight or whatever." Samantha described her nurse as "really nice. I could always call up if I had questions, and I had a lot of questions. She was really helpful. The whole staff there is really friendly. I mean they're excited when you're there and you're participating, so they're really gracious."

These once- or twice-daily shots required donors to inject a small needle into their stomachs or thighs. Women gave mixed reports about how much the shots hurt. Some said they "didn't really feel it," others described a "little pinch," and a few said the shots "can be painful, especially if you're on a schedule where you're taking several shots a day." It is very likely that a selection effect is at work here, because these women still decided to become egg donors even after they found out that it involves daily injections. Indeed, several made a point of saying that they are not scared of needles or that they have tattoos, so the prospect of giving themselves shots was not a "big deal."

The medications must be taken at the same time each day, and women reported slightly altering their schedules to do the injections. A few women hid the needles from people in their households. One of the younger donors, Valerie, a twenty-two-year-old college student, kept her entire first cycle a secret while living with her mother. This secret included the fact that she took her first-ever airplane trip to an out-of-state retrieval. Jane, just nineteen and in the midst of her third cycle, said her mother knew she was an egg donor but did not approve, so Jane tried to do the injections when she was not around. Susan, a twenty-four-year-old single mother, did not want to do the injections in front of her four-year-old, "because he doesn't understand that. That's weird to him, and so I'd do it before he got up." In addition to making time in their daily routines, several women changed other aspects of their behavior during cycles in response to requests from staff, including quitting smoking and reducing consumption of alcoholic beverages.

The injection of fertility medications stimulates the ripening of multiple eggs in the ovaries, a process that is monitored in physicians' offices through blood draws and ultrasound. Lisa, a twenty-six-year-old in the middle of her second cycle, described how the laboratory technician used ultrasound to view and count the ovarian follicles, which contain the ripening eggs. "They measured me. I was doing the injections for three days, and I went there on my fourth day before I took my fourth injection, and they found like six [eggs] on one [ovary] and seven on the other. They were still getting larger, and when I went today, they found a couple more. They had gotten a lot bigger since Wednesday. They develop quickly." Several donors thought it was "neat" to see their eggs, saying that they looked like "honeycomb" or "flowers." These visits are usually scheduled first thing in the morning, and, as a result, some women arrived late to work or had to arrange child care because commuting to the appointments took as much as an hour each way. Later in the day, women receive a call from the nurse if they need to adjust the dosage.

When the eggs are mature, donors do a final "trigger shot," which causes the ovaries to release the eggs. There was universal agreement that this injection is painful, as the medication goes in slowly and burns. Thirty-six hours later is the egg retrieval surgery, an outpatient procedure that usually lasts between fifteen and thirty minutes. In most cases, donors recall being prepped for surgery and then waking up in the recovery room. Dana, a twenty-five-year old who had donated four times in the past eighteen months, offers a fairly standard account of the day.

> You're up extremely early [*laughs*]. You can't have anything to eat the night before, which is horrible for me because I eat all the time. They put you in a room, have you undress, put on a hospital gown and a little cap to cover your hair. They start your IV and basically just let you sit for a while. They take your blood pressure, check your oxygen level, your saturation, your heart rate, make sure you go to the bathroom. They'll start some fluids and then wheel you into an OR. It's not the one you usually see in the hospital, but it's their version in their office. They get you on the bed, knock you out, and then that's it. You wake up, and you're back in the room you started in, and you really don't remember anything.

Women who donate to recipients who live elsewhere will often be asked to travel to the recipient's location for the last few days of the cycle. More than half the women I interviewed had traveled for at least one of their cycles. It is impossible to determine in advance the exact date of the retrieval, because it depends on how quickly the eggs mature, and this layer of uncertainty can add to the difficulty of scheduling time away from work and family. If an egg donor does have to travel, donation programs pay for one companion to join her on the trip, and several women considered this an opportunity to explore a new city with family or friends. Megan took her best friend along for a retrieval in the Northwest, saying, "I hadn't gone on a vacation in years," because she had been working full-time and taking a full load of classes at the university. Several Gametes Inc. donors had retrievals scheduled in Orlando, and they took their children along to go to Disney World, describing the trip as a "cheap family vacation." Other women preferred not to travel but had little choice because they lived in small towns. For example, Dana was a very popular donor who often had multiple recipients interested in her at the same time, so she would be asked where she preferred to donate. However, at the end of our interview, she concluded, "I don't mind the shots. I don't mind the appointments. I just don't like the travel [*laughs*]."

Side Effects

There are potential side effects from the fertility medications and the retrieval surgery (the details of which are discussed in the Introduction). Donors hear about these risks from program staff and psychologists as well as clinicians at the infertility practices where they are being treated. Before agreeing to donate, many women discussed these risks with relatives who were medical professionals or consulted their own doctors, and many did research online or in libraries.

As a result, egg donors are more than prepared to experience physical side effects. Of the seventeen women who had completed at least one cycle, eight described very mild reactions to the fertility medications and retrieval surgery, five experienced slightly more discomfort, and four described having serious pain.[6] On one end of the spectrum are almost breezy accounts, such as that offered by Erica, a twenty-seven-year-old mother of two who had donated twice in the previous year. "Really it's pretty simple [*laughs*]. You do a week or so of ultrasounds every day or every other day, depending on the medications, then go [*laughs*]. It's general anesthesia; you feel like you've slept for about four days, wake up feeling good. You just have light cramps for a couple days, and it's over and just back to normal life." Similarly, Jessica, a thirty-year-old nurse, explained,

> [Egg donation] really didn't take up a lot of time. The shots I did at home, and they just took a few minutes. It just didn't interfere with anything. I actually kept rollerblading and running and doing my regular things. I didn't have problems with it. They did say that you could have some cramping or bloating or just start to feel different things, and of course if you start to feel very odd, you should go see a doctor. I had a good experience with it, so it was just something that I kind of did and went on, and it never really bothered me, which I was glad. Up until the day we left [for the retrieval], that was actually the first day that I just started feeling like a little cramping feeling, and then for a couple days up until the retrieval and afterwards, but nothing that I can really speak of.

Jessica even referred to the retrieval as pleasant, noting, "Everybody was real nice, real pleasant. The doctor actually came in, introduced himself, and said 'This is what I'll be doing.' I was asleep through all of it anyway. I didn't get nervous. I was ready, just ready. It was a real pleasant experience."

For some women, recovery took no time at all, and they described going out for lunch or dinner after the retrieval. But others had cramping and bloating for a day or two. Jane explained how, as a result of the fertility medications, "you gain five pounds, which I think, if anything, is the part I hate most. You lose it after you get your period." Her cycle ended right before her sorority's formal dance. The discomfort from the injections made it difficult for her to practice the dance routine, and the extra weight made her feel self-conscious in her dress.

Olivia, a twenty-three-year-old who had completed three cycles, experienced more negative reactions to the fertility medications and the retrieval surgery but only in some of her cycles.

Olivia: The very first time I was fine. I didn't even think about it. I just took my shots every day. I thought, oh they're gonna take my eggs, and if she gets pregnant, yay, and if not, then at least I tried. I had no side effects. In fact, after the retrieval, I was up literally running around the office, because the nice head nurse Holly, she allowed me to go watch the retrieval of another woman. My mom had taken me out for lunch right after, I went home, watched TV, I was fine. The second time I did it [*laughs*] I was moody! I could be really happy one minute and then all of a sudden I would be like roar! Get out of my face!

Rene: Did they change the medication?
Olivia: Same medication. It's just your body responds differently different times. It's like a pregnancy. You never have the same pregnancy twice. I was moody, irritable, bloated. My stomach got all big. I had cramps. Bluh! It was horrible. I just went right home and was in bed for two days. And then the third time I was moody, no cramps, my tummy got big. They retrieve the eggs, and then it goes back to normal. I didn't have to go back to sleep or anything. I was fine.

Olivia was one of two women who reported not being given enough anesthesia during an egg retrieval. In describing the surgery for her third cycle, she said, "I won't say [it was] like someone stabbing you in your stomach, but if you could just imagine a big needle going into an area that's really tender and how much that would hurt and then the tender area being your ovaries." She was even awake enough to tell the doctor about the pain, but the procedure is so quick that there was not time to administer more anesthesia. However, this negative experience was not enough to deter her from donating again. She signed on for a fourth cycle, which just happened to be with the same physician. "I told the nurse, 'Next time, they're going to have to put me all the way under.'"

None of the egg donors I interviewed had severe reactions to the fertility medications or serious complications from the retrieval surgery, but on the far end of the side effects spectrum for this sample, four women (who were associated with three different donation programs) described experiencing a great deal of pain during the cycle. Moreover, "returning to normal" after the retrieval took a week or two instead of just a few days. Heather, who had just finished her first cycle, felt more pain as the cycle went on.

I went to [an ultrasound appointment] in the middle [of the cycle]. The [ovarian] follicles had gotten a lot bigger. That's when I started to actually feel my ovaries. It felt like cramps, not quite as uncomfortable. I was just very sluggish, almost bloated. Toward the end, like right before the surgery, it got really painful. Just sitting down kind of hurt because my ovaries were huge. There's like twenty-three enlarged follicles in my right one, and then in my left one, there were seventeen. [The nurse] described it to me: the ovaries sort of sag down a little bit because of all the weight and the fluid. I was like, "It makes so much sense now [*laughs*]." The ultrasound was the neatest part because you got to see everything growing, and I could feel everything that was going on. They were testing my hormone levels, and at the right stage, that night I take a trigger shot. Then I had a day off where it was pretty painful, so I just laid around. It wasn't like overbearingly painful. It was pretty much just cramps. It just felt like there were heavy ovaries.

Although most women reported producing between ten and twenty-five eggs during their cycles, the four donors who experienced more pain produced considerably more, between thirty and forty eggs. One woman said that after her first cycle, it "hurt to bounce or move too much" for several weeks, so she took matters into her own hands to ensure that she did not "overproduce" during subsequent cycles.[7]

My stomach was really distended. I was very uncomfortable. It was just not a good experience at all, so the second, third, fourth [cycles], I was very adamant about what I would and would not do. I would tell them, "You can't increase dosages on me, because I overproduce." The first time, I had thirty-three eggs, so then they knew we can't go this high. The second time, it went down to twenty-eight eggs. The third time, I started administering on my own, so it was like twenty-two. I had to take care of myself, and I know that's so against the rules. But they don't know how it goes for me. I just have to trust that my body is always going to react the same, which it does [*laughs*]. So it hovered around twenty-two the last two times, but that's still a lot of eggs. Some people, it's only like fourteen or ten. I would always start off, and they wouldn't be blossoming. By the tenth day, everything would go into overdrive. I didn't respond right away, so they're thinking they should step it up. They always err on the side of caution, which means get as many eggs as you can. So they would step it up from two ampoules to three, and that's when I didn't step it up. I didn't tell them. I just didn't do it. I hate saying this because if I really thought that I was wrong, then I wouldn't have done that because I wouldn't want anybody to be x'd out of their [chances for conceiving], but I couldn't go through the discomfort again. It's like you're pregnant, but you're not. It's just water, and it's hard. Even after the eggs are out, it doesn't go down right away.

Another donor who cycled multiple times with various agencies before taking a position as a staffer in an egg donation program echoed this suggestion that some physicians are more interested in generating eggs than in safeguarding donors' health. She explained that the same dose of medication affects women differently, but the number of eggs "also depends on the protocol the doctor uses. Some are a little more conservative than others, and there's a fine line between getting a good amount of eggs and hyperstimulating."

It is striking that three of the four women who experienced the most negative physical reactions went on to donate again, and the fourth wanted to have her own family first but would consider donating again in the future. Their subsequent cycles were much less painful, because physicians now knew to prescribe lower doses of medication. For example, Valerie's second cycle, which she described as "day" to the first cycle's "night," resulted in fifteen eggs instead of thirty-seven. In fact, the majority of egg donors—80%—were willing to do at least one more cycle, and many planned to donate several more times.[8] Nevertheless, several said there was a limit because of concerns they had about the effects of repeated exposure to fertility medications.

Aside from the four women on the far end of the side effects spectrum, Gretchen reported the most dramatic response to the shots. She was also the only person I interviewed who donated eggs to a close friend before signing up with a donation program. Her friend Barbara and her husband invited Gretchen to come live with them for the duration of the cycle, and given that Barbara had already tried IVF with her own eggs, she was in a position to tell Gretchen how it was going to go. Gretchen explained,

> Now Barbara was used to everything because she had already tried going through the cycle, so she knew what to expect, whereas me, I had no idea. I remember the first day of being on the Lupron as being horrible. I think it was just my body was not used to it. My hormones are going crazy. I was so nauseated I lived on popsicles for two days. I mean that's

all that I could stand. And then the second day, I remember getting a really bad headache. I think I popped two ibuprofen, and I was fine. But the funniest was when we were both on the Lupron. Their house is huge, and we kept cranking the air down lower and lower. Both Barbara and I would be walking through going, "God, is it like four hundred degrees in this house?" And her husband, bless his heart. Here we are in the middle of summer. It's like 95 degrees on a cold day up there. He's in jeans, a long-sleeved shirt, and a jacket, and he's like, "Are you kidding me?" He's like, "I can't put it down; you've got it set at 63. You need to suck it up and get past it." So that was the worst part about it.

It is possible that Gretchen was primed for this more dramatic response, because she was living with a woman who had already been through IVF once before trying to have a baby.

In fact, Lisa, whose forty-six-year-old mother was using IVF to have a family with her new husband, addressed this point explicitly. Here, she compares her experiences with fertility medications with those of women like her mother.

This particular drug I'm doing gives me a little bit of a red spot where I inject, but it just lasts for about a day. It's not that bad. The first time, I didn't have any side effects. No redness, nothing. I just felt normal. It was strange, because they kept sending me all this paperwork saying "This could happen, this could happen." But, no. They mentioned something about depression or euphoria, and I didn't really experience either. I think maybe that is more for people who are trying to get pregnant, because they're so nervous and desperate or whatever. They really want to get pregnant, and they get really emotional about it. I'm not really that emotional about it.

In sum, egg donors do not "live and die IVF." In stark contrast to infertile women, egg donors use straightforward, undramatic language to describe the injections and outpatient surgery and report that cycles are "easy" or "quick." Some women actually used the word "vacation" to describe traveling for the retrieval surgery, and even those who experienced more serious side effects went on to donate again. Although egg donors hope that recipients become pregnant, they are not nearly so invested in this outcome as infertile women are, because egg donors are not attempting their *own* long-awaited pregnancy. Moreover, they are paid thousands of dollars for the cycle, and they will receive the money regardless of how many eggs they produce. Perhaps this is the reason that so few women reference the financial compensation when discussing how egg donation fits into their daily lives. This is not at all the case with sperm donors, who, as will be clear in the next section, talk constantly about the money they make at the sperm bank.

THE EMBODIED EXPERIENCE OF SPERM DONATION

Whereas an egg donor is assimilated into a medical practice as a sort of patient, a sperm donor is required to perform a sexual act that has long been cloaked in shame and secrecy.[9] Few scholars have addressed the topic of masturbation, and some of the research that has been done has itself taken on an almost furtive quality. For example, in a landmark study of sexual behavior in the United States in 1992, Laumann and colleagues deemed questions about masturbation too sensitive to be asked out loud. Instead, the interviewer handed respondents a piece of paper with the questions listed, and respondents marked the answers before folding the paper, placing it in a sealed envelope, and handing it back to the interviewer.[10]

This survey revealed that more than 60% of men had masturbated in the last year, and about a third of the younger men (eighteen- to thirty-four-year-olds) reported doing it at least once a week. Selecting from a predefined list of reasons why they masturbate, men most commonly answered that they wished to relieve sexual tension or experience sexual pleasure. About half the men said they felt guilty about it. The researchers concluded that "masturbation has the peculiar status of being both highly stigmatized and fairly commonplace."[11] They distinguished it from sex with a partner and noted, "in this secluded personal realm, you do not have to pay as much attention to others, and the goal of personal pleasure can become central."[12]

Laumann and colleagues produced systematic statistics, but they did not collect qualitative data on the embodied experience of masturbation, a topic on which there has been very little research. In one study of Muslim men in Middle Eastern fertility clinics, Marcia Inhorn found that husbands, who must produce a semen sample timed to their wife's egg retrieval, experienced a great deal of anxiety, both from the need to perform and from violating religious mores. One man she interviewed explained, "In IVF centers, they say, 'Give me the sperm now! After five minutes, I need your sperm. Now, now! Give me, give me!' This is not good. The male encounters problems when they do that. It's not good. I start thinking about when I will give the sperm, and I feel uncomfortable." Pointing to the clinic's semen collection room, which had a door that opened into the small, crowded waiting room, this same man said it was "like a prison cell."[13] In some cases, the anxiety results in failure to produce a sample, and the IVF cycle is for naught.

Comparing the findings from Laumann et al.'s survey and Inhorn's interviews raises the question of how sperm donors experience masturbation. In the United States, the physical act is stigmatized, though not to the degree it is in the Middle East. Moreover, sperm donors are not masturbating on demand for a spouse in the next room who is undergoing complicated and expensive fertility treatments, but donors' payments are predicated on sperm count and semen volume. So do American men producing sperm for money experience masturbation more as paid pleasure or pressured performance?

From Awkward to Routine

Like the egg donors, the twenty sperm donors I interviewed were at various stages in the donation process, from those who had been making deposits for a few months to men who donated a decade before. Unlike the egg donors, none of the sperm donors mentioned being affiliated with more than one program, and all came from either Western Sperm Bank or Gametes Inc.[14] On average, men at Gametes Inc. had been producing samples for twenty-two months, compared to an average fifteen months at Western Sperm Bank (this comparison excludes one man at Gametes Inc. who had donated off and on for ten years, a very unusual length of time to be a donor). Most of the men—80%—were still actively donating. (More details about the interviews and the donors are available in the Introduction and appendixes.)[15]

Almost all the sperm donors described their first few visits to the bank as extremely awkward, but as they became acquainted with staff and developed familiarity with the procedures, donation became a routine part of their daily lives. Isaac, a twenty-two-year-old college student in a small Southeastern town, summarized transitioning from the "nerve-racking" first visit to getting "a little more comfortable with it."

> Coming back to actually donate and not just fill out paperwork was a little nerve-racking, because you got all these faces around that know exactly what you're about to do: walk in this bathroom and deposit into a plastic cup. It's a little unnerving. If you're not a very open or confident person, you could get easily embarrassed and scared out of it. My first couple times, I would always look in the parking lot, and thankfully there were no other donators coming in, so I knew it was just gonna be me. I'd do my thing, drop it off, and go. Nobody would see me except for [the program staff]. You think they won't be able to make eye contact, but it wasn't like that at all. This is what they do for a living. Basically, I guess it would be like your first day at a new job, except a little bit more uncomfortable. Even now when I'm in a rush, I feel like an idiot going in there, ten minutes later popping out, and dropping off my deposit. [The lab technician] once said to me, "Wow, Speedy Gonzales!" I'm like, "Yeah, well, I'm on a schedule." The impression they get of you sometimes can make you feel not as manly I suppose. I mean, it's gotten easier just to face everybody and go through it.

In describing his first deposit as akin to starting a "new job," except more "uncomfortable," Isaac is reflecting the sperm bank's framing of donation as a job as well as the cultural stigma around masturbation.

For some, the discomfort stemmed from religious beliefs. Manuel, a twenty-seven-year-old Christian living on the West Coast, was so embarrassed about donating that he did not tell his girlfriend for several months, even though they were living together. Here, he details a "transition" not unlike Isaac's, but for Manuel, his "upbringing" plays a role.

Manuel: There are just these booths, and it's not too much between your own privacy and what's on the outside, just that 1.5-inch piece of plywood.[16] In retrospect, it's not a big deal. It's just, coming from a Christian upbringing, it's like forbidden and taboo. This is doing something that would always have been just very—it felt bad! And I hate that feeling. Something is looking down and judging me for what I'm choosing to do. That's what I kind of felt at first. I didn't present that when I'm there. I'm nice, calm, cool. I'm in. I'm out. Take care of my business. No problem. No big deal. But in my mind, I'm thinking I've never done anything like this before. It's not like I'm a little kid, either. You'd think at a certain point I'd be more comfortable with it, but it wasn't that much easier. So if I tried it at like eighteen or nineteen, when I think they officially start to allow prospects, then it might have been even more uncomfortable.

Rene: So over the full year and a half [you donated], are you saying it never got any easier?
Manuel: It got easier. After maybe a few times, say three or four, it was just routine, because they were so accommodating, so nice, so receptive. At a certain point, I didn't feel uncomfortable at all. I think that was the whole point. In a way, we're doing a service, so they're going to want to make things as hospitable as they can, and they succeed very well, in my opinion. I don't know how it would be otherwise if it was very formal and impersonal. But it didn't feel like that, for the most part.

Rene: What would be "for the most part"? What was uncomfortable about it?
Manuel: Only if [the donor manager] wasn't there. When there's not a familiar face, that's when it would be a little different, sort of variation in the routine, but not to the point that it actually affected anything.

Rene: So how does [the donor manager] do that, take something that people find uncomfortable and turn it into this routine?
Manuel: She has a good personality. She has a good, sincere smile to her and a warm sort of nurturing mother feeling. That's how I felt with her. That might be looking too far into things. At the time, when I'm going through this, I'm not thinking all these things. I'm just doing it. She was always personable and asked me how I'm doing. It was one of those things where you develop a rapport with someone and that comes in time, of course, but she was like that from the beginning. I was probably the one who needed to make that transition more than

her. She's familiar with this. She's seen *how* many donors come and go? For me, it's not like I go to various sperm banks. It's not a routine for me. That was my transition.

Like Isaac, Manuel relies on the rhetoric of the workplace in that he "takes care of business" and defines potential donors as "prospects." This description also points to the importance of bank staff in shaping donors' experiences and establishing donation as routine. In fact, in my interview with the donor manager at Western Sperm Bank, she noted that when she took a vacation, she would often return to find that her "regulars" had stopped coming in. She would have to call them to get them back on schedule.

Once men do get in to a routine, donating sperm becomes just one more thing on the to-do list. Nathan, a thirty-eight-year-old who had started donating in his early twenties, explained how "you get into a rhythm, and you just think, oh it's Wednesday, I got to go down to Gametes Inc. Sometimes you forget. Two weeks go by. You have your lulls, or it just doesn't happen. You just find yourself putting it into your weekly schedule like getting groceries." Similarly, Greg, a college student, said that he might not make it to the bank if he had a test or if his motorcycle broke down. In general, though, he has "a schedule to come here. In my head I have to work it out. It's normally either on the way to or from school. So then I just try to figure out what I have to do today, how long I got to get it done, and then when I can fit this in."

Pleasure and Control

Upon arrival at most of the banks, men are buzzed in through secure doors, which is greater security than is in place at egg agencies. Sperm donors sign in and fill out a form with their donor number and answer questions about when they last ejaculated and whether they have had unprotected sex. Gametes Inc. had a new computerized check-in system that would automatically alert men when it was time to provide a urine sample or have their blood drawn. This needed to happen every few months so that the sperm samples could be released from quarantine and posted on the website for sale to recipients. Several men said that they did not look forward to blood draw day.

The donation rooms in each bank had slightly different décors. At CryoCorp, the founder proudly showed off what he called "masturbatoriums," small rooms with erotic pictures on the walls and flat-screen televisions for watching pornographic movies. Western Sperm Bank, a nonprofit, offered larger rooms with a small bed and chair but only provided magazines. Most of the sperm banks had several rooms so that more than one person could donate at a time, but University Fertility Services had a much smaller program, so men were simply directed to the clinic's bathroom, where there was a small stash of magazines in the drawer under the sink. Ethan, a thirty-nine-year-old who had just finished an eighteen-month stint at Western Sperm Bank, gave the most detailed description of the donation room and his routine.

> You go in a room, and they have a chair and a bed. It's comfortable, and they change the sheets, kind of like hospital linen. Even though it may not be clean, it always seemed to be smoothed out. And there's a big wicker basket full of sperm cups with a twist cap, and they're all individually hermetically sealed. A lot of times, they'll pick up one of those and set it in the middle of bed so it looks like no one's been there. It's like this nice hotel touch. First thing in the morning, it's always set up, but if they're really moving through people, especially later in the day, the pillow might be whatever, so you gotta kind of fluff the pillow. Or there might be a pubic hair on the bed. Sometimes I did masturbate thinking about my wife, but it wasn't the same. So I usually just grabbed a magazine to be sure that I would get aroused quick and get out of there. But in the beginning, it was kind of experimental and kind of fun. It was fun all the way through, actually. It became part of my day I enjoyed. It was like a stress release, and I got to look at really beautiful women without my wife going "I'm not letting you have a subscription to *Penthouse!*" [*laughs*] Guys were tearing—my favorite pictures would be gone some days, or your favorite magazine would disappear. You got used to your favorite room, because the rooms were decorated a little bit differently. I would get two magazines, especially if I knew them. This girl's really great, and this girl's really great, too. So I would lie down, and I would start masturbating. Then, at some point, you had to make a decision about how you were going to do this clinically. You have to sit up. I would have the cup sitting there, with the cap off and open, because if you were just about to

ejaculate and the cap wasn't off, you had to fumble. You could come all over yourself, and that's $50, a mess. I mean, it could be very embarrassing. It never happened to me. So you have to be conscious of that. It's not this free-flowing sexual activity.

In linking a spilled sample with $50, Ethan points to men's ever-present awareness of the fact that they are paid piece-rate.

About a third of the sperm donors echoed Ethan in saying that donation was pleasurable or fun, as it entailed an approved moment of looking at pornography and having an orgasm. Nevertheless, several agreed that this pleasure was constrained by the need to "stop and pay attention to that cup." Andrew, a twenty-eight-year-old graduate student, noted how in the sperm bank, masturbation is "not as pleasurable as it would be otherwise, because you have a little beaker thing and need to do a little more aiming [*laughs*]. I mean, still everything comes out, but it's not as good. You have to make sure everything's in the right place, as opposed to just kind of forgetting about it and letting everything go." He concluded by joking, "I get paid for it, so I make sacrifices."

Eighty percent of the sperm donors I interviewed exceeded the bank's minimum requirement of one deposit per week when they first started donating.[17] Most men need about forty-eight hours of abstinence to ensure a sperm count high enough to meet bank standards, so donating two or three times a week required refraining from sexual activity for four to six days out of every seven. Many of the men engaged in experiments to see how little abstinence they needed or, in the words of one donor, "how my body worked." Manuel reported that he could pass samples with just thirty-six hours of abstinence. Dennis, who had been donating for eleven months and was weary of his commitment to the bank, used to donate once every three days but had cut back to just once a week and still only passed some of his samples.

In detailing his donation schedule, Isaac pointed out that the amount of time he spent *preparing* to donate was much greater than the actual amount of time he spent inside the bank.

I try to make three times a week: Monday, Wednesday, Friday. Basically that means Monday, if I get here in the morning, then I have approximately six to twelve hours to enjoy life with my fiancée [*laughs*]. Then I have to be abstinent for the next day and a half, normally about thirty-eight to forty, thirty-six to forty-four hours, something like that to be prepared for Wednesday to deposit. Then Friday, I have a nice long day. Saturday about halfway through the day, I gotta be abstinent again. I mean really the biggest pain is probably the abstinence thing. Not because it's lack of sex or anything. It's just because this takes like fifteen, twenty minutes out of your day, not including time driving, probably thirty, forty minutes depending on where you live. It's cool; you get paid a nice little chunk of money for basically three hours a week. But you're actually working quote unquote like a whole forty-hour week because you have to abstain. You have to make sure you're not doing anything wrong and especially trying to get enough sleep and all that and not getting too stressed, because that can affect the count.

Indeed, the issue of abstinence came up in almost all of my interviews with sperm donors, which probably reflects the need to regulate their sexual activity for such a long period of time. In contrast, very few egg donors mentioned it at all, even though women must refrain from sexual contact for several consecutive weeks because of the high risk of pregnancy associated with fertile women taking fertility drugs.[18]

Many sperm donors echoed Isaac's complaints, and it was especially those men in serious relationships who groused about having to "schedule" their sex lives. Scott, a thirty-two-year-old who is married with three children, said that "from a personal standpoint, you have to stay on a schedule, which at times is a little frustrating. There's a lot of times when your body isn't set up to, I mean you kind of go through moods, regardless of what that schedule is going to be. There are times when it's: uhh I can't, not tonight."

Some men held firm to the schedule, but others would occasionally skip visits to the bank. Kyle, a twenty-two-year-old who lived with his girlfriend explained,

Every now and then, she has rolled over in the middle of the night. I know I have to come [to the sperm bank] the next day, and she wants to [make love], and I'm thinking to myself that's $100. Sometimes I do, and I'm like, "Are you going to pay me $100 like they do?" Sometimes I don't. I say, "Well, we have this to pay for." But it's not a stressful thing. I like it, too, because when we do make love, it's once a week, probably twice a week, and it's just on Friday and Saturday, so it makes it a little better because of the anticipation. She don't complain, because she knows that if she wants that nice couch and the nice bedroom furniture and the nice place, I gotta keep coming here. But it doesn't bother me at all.

Like Kyle, Ryan, a forty-year-old who had been donating once a week for the last several years, referenced the money in discussing how he smoothed over the issue of abstinence with his wife, calling it a "peace offering."

None of the egg donors mentioned male partners complaining about abstinence, but several sperm donors talked about how their girlfriends or wives would occasionally get annoyed at having to adhere to a schedule. Ethan and his wife would only have sex on Fridays, an arrangement that did not make her happy, so they tried having sex without climax. But then Ethan's samples stopped passing. He talked to the donor manager, who told him, "You can't have your cake and eat it, too. You have to abstain."

Other than failing to abstain, donors reported a long list of reasons why their samples might not pass the bank's strict requirements: being tired or stressed, getting sick, exercising right before donating, working outside in hot weather, drinking too much alcohol, eating poorly, smoking marijuana, and hot-tubbing. Charles, a twenty-nine-year-old graduate student who had donated sporadically for the last five years, noted, "if I haven't been eating exactly as I should have or if I haven't been getting enough sleep, I can tell my body isn't ready to donate. After a while, you kind of get a feel for when you're ready, and sometimes I just don't feel up to it."

If men had several failing samples in a row, bank staff sometimes inquired if anything had changed or offered pointers. Most donors found this advice helpful and altered their behavior, which included taking vitamins and other supplements, drinking more orange juice, eating more protein, or reducing alcohol consumption. Greg, a college student who donated twice a week, said he started drinking more beer over the summer and as a result was only passing 25% to 50% of his samples. He asked a donor friend as well as the donor manager and the bank's physician how to improve his pass rate, and, in response to their advice, was "changing a lot of my eating habits and a lot of my other habits so I can get more money [*laughs*]."

In sum, sperm donors certainly do not experience the deep anxiety of men producing samples for their wives' fertility treatments. But their embodied experiences also do not conform to Laumann et al.'s description of masturbation as occurring in a "secluded personal realm" where "personal pleasure" is central.[19] Walking into a sperm bank requires that men overcome the stigma of masturbation, produce a semen sample in a small room, and then hand over the plastic cup to a lab technician, who will run tests to determine whether he will get credit for that deposit. Outside the bank, sperm donors must maintain bodily control, not only in terms of sexual activity, but also in terms of eating, drinking, and sleeping. So although men do derive some pleasure from the "sexual release," it is just one small part of what is involved in being a paid sperm donor.

CONCLUSION

Women and men who are paid to produce sex cells must manage their own bodies: women through shots and surgery and men through routine masturbation and abstinence. Although they have very different physical experiences of gamete donation, both egg and sperm donors provide evidence that variation in social context is associated with variation in bodily experience. Egg donors describe the injections and egg retrieval in much less onerous terms than do infertile women, because being paid thousands of dollars and not trying to become pregnant results in a different embodied experience of IVF. Sperm donors portray masturbating for money as requiring a surprising amount of bodily discipline while rendering the orgasm less pleasurable, which leads them to make distinctions between their embodied experiences of masturbation inside and outside the sperm bank.

For some, these findings will make intuitive sense. After all, there is enormous heterogeneity in all kinds of bodily experiences. But there is a strong assumption, among both scholars and clinicians, that IVF is inherently difficult and demanding, an assumption that derives in part from a well-developed feminist critique of the technology.[20] For example, anthropologist Monica Konrad interviewed British egg donors and was shocked to find that they described donation as "simple" and "quick." Even after she read to them from a pamphlet describing the shots and surgery, she was "struck by [the donors'] reluctance to comment in any detail on certain aspects of the egg induction process. To an outsider, the process seemed an exceptional commitment, if not an onerous and risky undertaking." In the end, Konrad steps in with her own assessment when she writes that the donors "*downplay* the considerable amount of preparation time that must be invested in the process" and are "*refusing* to acknowledge the pain, discomfort, and risk."[21] Rather than dismissing egg donors' statements, I suggest another explanation for why their descriptions do not conform to researchers' expectations, namely that their embodied experiences of the technology *are* different from the infertile women who are most often the subject of research on IVF.

Social scientists have focused on the many ways in which people "see" the body or "think" about the body, but the experiences of gamete donors contribute to a growing literature that suggests there is also variation in how the body *feels*.[22] Some studies have begun to examine particular mechanisms through which the "social" manifests in the material body, with social factors including everything from individual experiences to structural inequalities. For example, stress results in physiological damage, major life events (such as divorce or the death of a spouse) increase the probability of illness, and relative class status may result in different levels of mortality.[23] In the medical market for sex cells, it is the social process of commodification that influences women's and men's embodied experiences of donation.

FOUR **Being a Paid Donor**

Producing eggs and sperm involve very different physical processes, but the women and men who apply to be donors are very similar in one regard: most are drawn in by the prospect of being paid. In egg agencies, though, staffers draw on gendered cultural norms to talk about the money as compensation for giving a gift, yet sperm bank staffers consider payments to be wages for a job well done. Given that egg and sperm donors are walking in the door for similarly pecuniary reasons, what happens when they encounter the organizational framing of paid donation as a gift or a job?

By the organizational framing of paid donation, I mean the constellation of gendered practices and rhetorics in egg agencies and sperm banks that are detailed in Chapter 2, which include the amount of attention given to the donor/recipient relationship and the different payment protocols. Women are paired with a specific recipient, and the donation involves a relatively brief but focused period of time in which the donor takes shots, attends medical appointments, and has her eggs retrieved. Thus, even when egg donors do not meet recipients, the idea that someone is on the other end of the exchange is more present, both because staffers talk about recipients more and because women know that their eggs are going to a specific person who has chosen them. In contrast, sperm donors do not hear much about recipients and are not allowed to meet them. Men are also donors for a much longer period of time during which they make routinized deposits at the bank, more like employees clocking in and out on a regular basis. The underlying message conveyed by these organizational practices, that donation is a gift or a job, is reinforced by payment policies: egg agencies disburse a lump sum at the end of the cycle regardless of how many eggs a woman produces, while sperm banks cut a check every two weeks—but only for those samples that meet bank standards.

There are countless sociological studies about how events or interactions are "framed" in different ways.[1] However, less is known about what happens when organizations rely on different kinds of frames for similar kinds of activities, particularly in terms of how such variation affects the individuals who are involved with those organizations. Kieran Healy has addressed this question in cross-national research on blood and organ donation. He found that donation programs "create and sustain their donor pools by providing opportunities to give and by producing and popularizing accounts of what giving means."[2] Healy did not conduct qualitative research with donors though, so his finding raises new questions. Does "what giving means" change depending on the bodily good being donated, especially if those goods are more associated with male bodies or female bodies? Moreover, how do donors respond to an organization's gift rhetoric when they are also receiving direct payments? These are pressing questions for scholars of bodily commodification, because there has been so much concern about the dehumanizing effects of being paid for parts of one's body.

In this chapter, I look at how women and men who produce sex cells respond to the organizational framing of paid donation, finding that it *does* have consequences for how individuals experience bodily commodification. Despite the fact that egg and sperm donors are alike in being motivated by the compensation, and they spend the money on similar things, they end up adopting gendered conceptualizations of what it is they are being paid to do. Women speak with pride about the huge gift they have given, while men consider donation to be a job, and some sperm donors even reference feelings of alienation and objectification.

"I'M IN IT FOR THE MONEY"

The vast majority of egg and sperm donors I interviewed revealed that their initial interest in donation was sparked by the prospect of financial compensation, which is understandable given their life circumstances.[3] Most were working but were doing so in low-paying jobs that were often part-time (see Table 2). Moreover, about half the donors were also students, including those who were taking a few classes at the local junior college and those who were enrolled full-time at a four-year university. Of those who were not employed at the time of the interview, three women were students who worked in the service sector before donating eggs, one woman was a librarian who now takes care of her young children, and the three men were students whose primary financial support came from fellowships or family members.

Table 2   Egg and Sperm Donors' Occupations

	Women (n=19)	Men (n=20)
Service sector	3	6
Clerical work	8	3
Manual labor	0	1
Education / Health / Firefighting	3	2
Salaried professional	1	5
Not employed	4	3

Given the low wages of service and clerical work as well as students' perennial need for money, the prospect of earning thousands of dollars for providing sex cells exerts a strong pull. Megan, a twenty-two-year-old who went to school full-time while also holding down a full-time job as a clerk, said "I would fail out of school sometimes because I had to work so much." After hearing Creative Beginnings' advertisement on the radio, she emailed to ask for more information. She explained,

> What came in the mail was just their poster. It said what they did, the opportunity to earn up to $5,000, so it would just seem like a lot of money to me. I've never had a lot of money all at once. It said anonymity guaranteed. It had photos of women who were young and my age and doing this type of thing. Sporty! [*laughs*] Then it has pictures of happy husbands and wives, brand new babies. It was really, really good marketing.

Later in the interview, she added that "it wasn't a terrible amount of money. It wasn't so much that it was irresistible. It was something that I chose to do, because it could help someone else." Exhibiting a similar ambivalence about being too focused on the compensation, Gretchen, a recent college graduate, said "This is what makes me feel like a horrible person: I'm in it for the money. Honestly, my car is going to die. The boost in income is going to be nice."

Men are not so reluctant to identify their primary interest in donation as monetary. Manuel, an undergraduate with a part-time library job when he began donating in his mid-twenties, explained, "As a student, I was thinking of which ways to make ends meet financially. That's the bottom line. How can I make money without really getting a second job? Then you hear about things like sperm donation, so I looked it up on the Internet. My first step was just calling and finding out what kind of pay do you get? What do I need to do to make this happen? There was no desperation. I wasn't hard up for money. This [library] job only pays so much, and the extra money could help."

Dennis, a recent graduate of a prestigious university, did describe himself as somewhat desperate. He was living with roommates and working at several part-time jobs when he finally decided to respond to a Western Sperm Bank ad he had seen many times before.

Looking for jobs on [the website] Craigslist once a month, maybe twice a month, [the sperm bank] puts up an ad that says, "Making money never felt so good."[*laughs*] It's really corny. I kept seeing it, and I was really strapped for cash, so I looked into it. [After-school teaching] was only twelve hours a week, $8 an hour. Not enough to live on. I needed to do something else, so I started SAT tutoring. I just applied for a ton of stuff at the same time.

Later in the interview, he filled in a little more detail about what this "ton of stuff" entailed. "At the time, I was trying to get into medical studies. I really needed cash. I was willing to sell my body, anything, sperm, whatever. I was trying to get into a study for opiate addicts. If there was money involved, I would do it. It's just my body. It'll heal, whatever they do to it [*laughs*]. It's a party body."

About a third of the donors, including Dennis, took care to mention that their monetary interests were not so strong that they felt the need to whitewash their profiles, especially in terms of reporting their family's health history. Heather, a college student, was worried that she would not be accepted as a donor because her "father died of a heart attack, and so did his parents. I was like, 'Oh there's a big negative sign there.' But I put it down anyways, because if I lie about that sort of thing and then later on down the road this child develops something, I couldn't lie about that. It's important. So I would rather have them not pick me up than lie about that."

For other donors, this impulse only went so far. One of the younger women agreed that it was important to be truthful in regard to family health history but not necessarily in other parts of the profile.

I tried to answer everything [on the profile]. Some of the things, you kind of tell little fibs. How often do you drink? It's like, come on! [*laughs*] I really wanted a match, and so I said I drink less than I really do. I used to smoke. So I tried to be honest about that, because I thought maybe that would be a concern. [The donor manager] looked at my profile, and she said, "Can you quit? I don't accept donors that smoke." I was like, "Okay I'll quit." Just little things. Have you ever tried recreational drugs? Hello, who hasn't?! [*laughs*] But as long as I'm not doing it while I'm in the cycle, then I think it should be okay. The part about my family [history], I had to force the information out of my parents, about when were [relatives] born, when did they die, how much did they weigh. [My parents said,] "Why are you asking all these questions?" [I told them,] "It's for a project at school." With all my aunts and uncles, I don't really know all the diseases and stuff. I know that if somebody had something in my family, my parents would have told me, so with that, of course to the best of my knowledge, I tried to be as truthful as possible.

In another case, an egg donor, who is herself a woman of color, had encouraged several Asian American friends to donate, because she knew they were "in demand." In response to a question about whether she gave her friends any advice about filling out the profile, she paused before explaining,

> Some of my friends were complaining about how they didn't get matches. I told them, "Just say you're Chinese." [laughs] Yeah, because I think Asian features, they're all alike. A lot of couples want pure Chinese, so it kind of sucks. [My friends] want to get matched. They are Chinese, they're like maybe half Chinese, but they're still Chinese.

These kinds of reports were not common in the interviews, but the potential for this sort of subterfuge exists, because there is no way of independently verifying most of the information that donors provide on profiles.

"HELPING OTHERS"

About a fifth of the donors started out with a very different motivation: they were primarily interested in helping recipients have children. In comparison to donors who were "in it for the money," these donors were at a different point in their lives, more likely to be married, to have children, and to be financially comfortable. All five sperm donors in this category were salaried professionals, and all started donating at older ages. The three egg donors were a little more heterogeneous in terms of employment; one was a music teacher, another was a housewife, and the third occasionally worked in part-time clerical positions.

The donors who signed on to help others were also more likely to be close with someone who had experienced infertility. Lisa, a twenty-six-year-old mother of two young children, decided to become a donor when she learned that her mother was using IVF to start a new family. "I have a tubal ligation, and I don't want any more kids. I figure I'm young, and I'm making good eggs. I might as well give them to somebody who could use them. I'm just kind of a philanthropic person anyway. I like to donate money or clothes or what have you to different organizations. This is just kind of like the ultimate gift you can give to somebody."

Two donors had experienced infertility in their own marriages. After having three children with her husband, Rosa had a tubal ligation in her early twenties. However, when he died in a car accident, she remarried and went through almost two years of medical procedures to have a child with her new husband. Rosa described flipping through a magazine while waiting for an optometrist's appointment with her children when an ad "popped up" at her, asking, "Do you want to help a family that can't have children?" She called the egg agency, and over the course of the next several years, she twice donated eggs and once served as a surrogate mother.

Evincing a similar empathy, Ryan, a forty-year-old engineer whose wife had difficulty conceiving their daughter, decided to switch from being a regular blood donor to being a regular sperm donor.

> We knew that [my wife] had some previous problems and maybe couldn't get pregnant. She did actually get pregnant shortly after we got married, but it was a miscarriage. We tried later and had a little girl. I just started thinking about it, the joy, the loss of our child, and not being able to have a child. I understand what some of these couples might be going through, but I also understood when a miracle does happen. That's kind of why I decided to do [sperm donation], just to kind of help others. To be honest, the money from the little donation does help out, and we decided we'd use it toward my daughter's [education fund]. So every check we get, we deposit it into that account.

Being interested in helping recipients does not preclude appreciating the income from donation. Ryan was a well-paid engineer not in need of the extra cash, but in referring to how he "helps others" while the money "helps out" his family, he suggests a mutualism to donation.

Three of the men are single professionals without children who referenced a slightly different version of "helping": they wished to make their genes available to recipients as an act of charity. Travis, a thirty-year-old engineer, pointed out that he had a large family filled with relatives who lived long, healthy lives. So he considered giving "amazing genes" to "people who are trying to have kids" as just one of his many philanthropic endeavors alongside blood donation and community service projects. Ben, a twenty-six-year-old software engineer, invokes not only health and longevity, but also intelligence and athleticism.

Ben: I think I have something to contribute. I feel like I'm a very intelligent individual. I come from a family of very bright people, and we're all athletic. We live very long lives, very healthy. We don't have any really serious issues until we're in our eighties and nineties. I thought that I'm just a prime candidate for donating sperm, and I'd like to be charitable. I give a lot of my money to charitable organizations. I really don't like donating blood. I like to keep that part to myself. Anybody can really do a lot of these things, but not very many people can donate sperm. So I thought that I'd really be adding something to the community if I did that. So that's really [it]. Because I'm independently wealthy, I'm not interested in the money. I don't even accept the money that they give. I give it to my brother who's a postdoc with a wife and kids.

Rene: So, all the way back in high school, what made you respond positively [to the idea of sperm donation]? Was it just you're smart and you felt like you could contribute this?
Ben: Absolutely. I thought that if there were more people like me in the world, the world would be a little better, not by that much, a tiny, little, hardly significant amount, but I'd have contributed positively. There's not very many things as an individual to contribute positively, and this was one of them.

Later in the interview, I asked Ben, "Of all the charitable things you could do, why is this important for you?" He replied, "Because I believe very strongly that our genes are a large part of who we are, and I think I've been blessed with a very strong, very good genetic heritage, and I feel like other people should be blessed."[4]

For most men, the sperm bank was nearby, on the way to work or school, so donating did not involve going more than five or ten minutes out of the way. But three of the men who signed on to help others made much longer trips. Scott drove ten miles from work to the bank, saying, "I can round-trip it in forty-five minutes, so it works for a lunch break." Ryan drove twenty-five miles each way, and Ben commuted an hour each way. Scott and Ryan are also among the longest-serving donors, at thirty and thirty-three months, respectively. This suggests that their commitment to helping people is strong enough to survive not only these lengthy commutes, but also the need to regulate their sexual activities for such a long period of time.

EARNING AND SPENDING

Given that so many donors are motivated by the money, it is important to look closely at what women and men actually earn from paid donation. As noted in Chapter 2, commercial egg agencies often pay different rates to different donors, with first-timers receiving around $5,000 per cycle, a number that will generally increase for additional cycles or for women with particularly sought-after characteristics. University-based programs usually pay less, sometimes as little as $2,000 per cycle.

Egg donors reported fees for forty-one cycles that occurred between 1998 and 2006. The fees ranged from $2,000 to $10,000 per cycle with an average payment of $4,297. Of the thirteen women who had donated more than once, five were paid more for additional cycles, five were paid the same, and three were paid less (see Table 3).[5] Women in metropolitan areas occasionally donated through multiple programs, which explains some of the variation in compensation (cycles at programs other than those where I did research are italicized in the table).

In each of the commercial agencies, there was at least one woman whose fee increased, though it was less common at Gametes Inc., where

Table 3 Compensation per Cycle for Women Donating Multiple Times[*]

Donor	Program	Years	Cycle #1	Cycle #2	Cycle #3	Cycle #4	Cycle #5	Cycle #6	Cycle #7
			FEES INCREASED						
Nicole	OvaCorp	1998–1999	$3,000	$3,500	$4,000	$5,000			
Beth	OvaCorp	1999–2002	$3,500	$4,000	$4,500	$10,000	$6,000	$5,000	$8,000
Lisa	OvaCorp	2002	$4,000	$6,000					
Jane	Creative Beginnings	2002	$6,500	$5,500	$8,000	$8,000			
Dana	Gametes Inc.	2005–2006	$3,500	$5,000	$5,000	$5,000	$7–8,000		
			FEES UNCHANGED						
Samantha	Creative Beginnings	2001–2002	$4,000	$4,000					
Erica	Gametes Inc.	2006	$5,000	$5,000					
Pam	Gametes Inc.	2006	$5,000	$5,000					
Susan	Gametes Inc.	2006	$5,000	$5,000					
Valerie	Gametes Inc.	2006	$5,000	$5,000					
			FEES DECREASED						
Rosa	OvaCorp	1998–1999	$2,500	$1,500					
Olivia	Creative Beginnings	2000–2002	$5,000	$5,000	$3,000				
Gretchen	University Fertility Services	2006	$5,000	$2,000					

[*] "Program" refers to the donation program through which I contacted the donor. Cycles that are in italics took place at other programs. In Olivia's case, she had not yet completed a cycle at Creative Beginnings.

staff does not routinely offer higher fees. In Samantha's case, Creative Beginnings does generally pay more, but she donated a second time to a couple who did not become pregnant the first time, so this may have prevented staff from asking for a higher fee. Of those whose fees declined, Rosa's second cycle was cancelled before the egg retrieval, so she was only given a partial fee. Olivia donated through two commercial agencies before signing on with a university program, which paid less per cycle. Gretchen donated to a friend before signing up with University Fertility Services, where she was paid $3,000 less, a difference she thought was "logical," because "if you know somebody, of course they're going to pay you more." She was "disappointed" that the university paid so much less.[6]

In most cases, program staffers determine the fee, and egg donors are not always aware of the reasoning involved. For example, Lisa, a twenty-six-year-old, was told by OvaCorp's donor manager that the "first time around, they usually pay 3,000 [dollars]." So she was surprised when the higher "price" of $4,000 appeared on her first contract in 2002. "For some reason, [the donor manager] asked for more money for me from this first couple. I think it was because I had already had two children and my age. She said I was desirable." When I asked Lisa what that meant, she responded with a laugh, "Good eggs, I don't know, good genes." Likewise, Kim, another OvaCorp donor who was a twenty-three-year-old college graduate, did not know why she was being paid $5,000 for her first cycle but joked, "I'm not going to complain."

In two cases, the request for a higher fee came from the donor, and it is worth noting that Jane and Dana ended up with some of the highest fees in the sample. Dana did not make this request until her fifth cycle, when she and the Gametes Inc. donor manager decided to ask for $8,000 from the recipients, who countered with $7,000. The negotiation was ongoing at the time of our interview. Like other egg donors, Dana expressed ambivalence about focusing on the money. "I've really felt bad about asking for that much. I didn't want to feel greedy, but at the same time, as much as you have to go through, not only physically but mentally, and the time you have to take away from your job and your family, you really need to be compensated for it."[7]

There is much less variation in what men are paid per donation, with most banks offering the same flat rate to all donors. This was set at $50 at the nonprofit Western Sperm Bank and $75 at the for-profit CryoCorp in 2002. Gametes Inc. has a two-tiered system, paying anonymous donors $65 and identity-release donors $100 per sample in 2006. But even these slight differences in rates combine with variation in how often men donate to create a wide range of earnings among sperm donors. Staffers encourage men to make weekly deposits (at least), but some donors choose to donate two or three times a week. It is very common for samples not to pass, though. So men who make $50 per sample and donate (and pass) one sample each week will make $200 in a month, and those who make $100 per sample and donate (and pass) three samples each week can make as much as $1,200 in that time.

Inevitably, sperm banks trumpet the highest amount possible in their advertisements, but donors rarely achieved this level of income on a regular basis. Four men who were paid $50 per sample at Western Sperm Bank reported earning between $250 and $500 per month (average: $375). Seven identity-release donors who were paid $100 per sample at Gametes Inc. reported earning between $600 and $1,200 per month (average: $930). Moreover, an individual donor's earnings could fluctuate quite a bit from month to month. For example, Victor, a twenty-three-year-old identity-release donor at Gametes Inc. referred to himself as a "full-time donor" because he makes three deposits each week. "Usually my samples make it. Sometimes I may have had a bad week, and two samples didn't make it. So, I'm saying anywhere from $360 to $540 every two weeks." Victor's calculations are based on multiples of $90, because Gametes Inc. is the only program to withhold $10 from each passing sample as an incentive to the donor to show up for periodic blood tests. If the donor passes the tests, the accumulated money is disbursed.

About half the women who lived in metropolitan areas applied to multiple programs, either to increase their chances of being chosen by a recipient or because they were rejected by the first program they contacted. Sperm donors were less likely to engage in this behavior both because there are fewer sperm banks and because of the more intensive time commitment. For example, Andrew, who was in graduate school, did look into another program that was about forty-five minutes away. That program paid $75 or $100 compared to the $45 he received when he first signed on with Western Sperm Bank, but he did not want donation "to be a huge time commitment. Western Sperm Bank is close to where I work, so I can stop in a couple times a week and work it around my work schedule."

Just as egg and sperm donors express similar motivations for donation, they spend the money on similar things. It is "special money," in that it is earmarked for particular purposes; just 5% of the donors did not have a specific plan for it.[8] A few donors, including two divorced mothers of young children and four single men working multiple low-wage jobs, did use the money to cover basic living expenses. But most donors did not portray their financial situations in such dire terms. About half used at least some of the money to pay off debt, as did Dana.

> The first time I had a retrieval, I was only paid $3,500, and I used it to pay off bills [*laughs*]. I'd gotten out of college and didn't have anything, so I had to buy furniture, this and that, and I got it all on credit. So I just paid a lot of that off and then bought stuff for my house that I own now. Every other time since, I've gotten 5,000 [dollars]. [The second retrieval] was paying off some more bills and just kind of doing stuff around the house. [The third retrieval] was to pay off Disney World tickets [*laughs*] that I put on my credit card, and I bought a vehicle. I put a big down payment on an [SUV]. The [fourth retrieval], I paid off bills from my wedding [*laughs*]. So, I've really accomplished a lot with the money.

Egg donors were more likely to use at least some of the money for school, either by paying for tuition or by paying off student loans. Samantha worked full-time as a clerk while also going to college. She attended a community college for two years before transferring to a state university, where she took twenty credits per quarter and went to summer school in order to graduate in one year. The money from egg donation was "exciting because that would go toward school. I'm trying to pay for school myself, so that was like a really big help. I just put it in savings, and I didn't really touch it. Then, each quarter, when they send the billing account, I'd take from it and pay for it that way. When I was almost done with school, which wasn't too long ago, then I put the rest, almost, not all of it, the rest toward my car." Budgeting such large payments is probably made easier by the fact that egg donors' compensation comes in the form of one lump sum.

In contrast, sperm donors are paid every few weeks, and they were more likely to classify the money as "expendable income." For example, Fred, a fraternity brother, used it to buy alcohol and food on weekends. Paul, another undergraduate, put what he earned from his other part-time jobs into savings and directed the money from sperm donation to "groceries and gas and usually a little something extra, a shirt or something every few weeks." Just one of the sperm donors diverted the money to educational expenses. Either men's parents paid for school, or they qualified for a state scholarship.

Several of the younger women and men suggested that earning money as donors made them more financially responsible. Mike, a twenty-two-year-old with credit card debt from when he was a teenager, described paid donation as "a way for me to be that guy that always pays his bills. It's just helped me grow and become more responsible as a person, rather than just sitting around, scrounging around for money, trying to get it waitering or doing whatever else I'd have to do to make it. It's just makes me more financially responsible." Jane, the daughter of financially struggling immigrants and a student at a prestigious university, had already completed three cycles with Creative Beginnings before turning twenty. She said, "Being an egg donor, I'm earning my own money. I'm trying to take care of myself. It makes me a little more independent."

Donors who were initially motivated by the idea of helping recipients were more likely to save the money from donation or use it to buy extras for themselves or their families. Lisa, a music teacher, described the money from egg donation as "gravy." She used the fee from her first cycle to buy a vintage car, which she planned to repaint with the fee from her second cycle. Travis, an engineer with an MBA who was not dating anyone at the time, kept his earnings in a special "kitty." He said that his family was both religious and conservative, and he had not disclosed his activities at the sperm bank to them. His own ambivalence about the money and how he was making it is evident in how he managed it.

Travis: I cash the checks, don't put them in the bank, and I just put them in this thing. I use a little bit for extra cash from time to time, but by and large, I'm just kind of saving it right now. I've thought about different things. Well whenever I get married or engaged, I'll use that money to buy an engagement ring. So it's kind of like—I don't want to say turning the bad to good—but kind of like using something that wasn't, that was for something else. What am I gonna do with this money every week? I don't want to have nothing at the end of the day or year that I've got to show for this. I'll just put it away and use it for something. I don't know what.

Rene: *That's so interesting because you're an MBA, and you would presumably know everything about accounting, that you would have a little, almost Depression Era—*
Travis: [*laughs*] Exactly. With every other penny I make with my regular income, I have investments and planning, and I own a house and all this stuff. I've got all that allocated, and that's why with this, it's just kind of hiding money under the mattress. Everything else is so structured. This has no purpose, no direction. This is just a little savings stockpile, rainy day, something. I mean, I've got rainy day money, but this is just kind of different. I don't know.

Rene: *Do you know how much is in there?*
Travis: No, I have no idea.

Scott, a married professional, categorized the income from sperm donation as "just play money," which he spends on extras for his three kids.

It doesn't generally even hit the books the same way. I mean the other [paychecks from our jobs], automatically in, and we've already got it set up to pay bills. Overall household income, [the money from sperm donation] doesn't impact it that much, but it does give us a little extra so that we can do the stuff that we want to do with the kids: Six Flags season passes. That kind of stuff we wouldn't be able to do if we didn't have that.

Donors who treated themselves were generally single without children, and those who bought extras for others were usually in serious relationships and/or had children.

BEING PAID TO GIVE A GIFT OR PERFORM A JOB

Women and men sign on to donate for similar reasons, and they spend the money on similar things, so it would follow that they would talk about this activity—being paid to produce sex cells—in similar ways. But in fact, this is not the case. Women portray donation as a gift, while men consider it a job, rhetorical variation that maps directly onto the gendered organizational framing of donation in egg agencies and sperm banks.

Donors' trajectories, from their initial interests in donation to how they come to define what kind of activity it is, are presented in stylized form in Figure 4.[9] The few donors whose initial interest was sparked by the prospect of helping recipients have children remain committed to this goal. However, those who were initially motivated by money eventually adopt different ways of conceptualizing donation, with women making use of gift rhetoric and men relying on employment rhetoric.[10] Only one man called donation a gift, and just three women said it was a job. Two of these three women did so while explaining how they originally thought of donation as a job but now think about it in terms of helping recipients.

Throughout the donation process, as women interact with staff, and occasionally with recipients, they hear over and over that egg donation is a gift. In fact, women often encounter this framing in their very first contact with programs, either through advertisements or through conversations with donor managers. Kim, a recent college graduate whose "whole intention of getting this extra money is getting out of debt," had been matched with a recipient, but she had not yet donated. I asked when she first learned about the compensation.

> Well, of course right up front. The way [OvaCorp's donor manager] explains it, it's so cute. "It's a gift; it's a gift" [*singing and laughing*]. She's like, "You're giving a gift, and you just deserve to get something in return for it." It sounds so not like, I guess when you just think of it, it's just ah I'm getting money, but she makes it sound like it's a gift. Very cute.

Describing a similar message from Creative Beginnings, Megan went to the donation program's information session thinking "the biggest

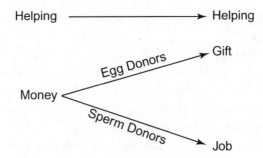

Figure 4. Donors' initial interests in and
current conceptualizations of paid donation

[stereotype] for me was that you could do [egg donation] as many times
as you wanted to, that you could profit on basically selling body parts.
At the meeting, I learned it's more like a blood donation and a Good
Samaritan deed."

The recipient of this gift does not remain an abstraction, because staffers regularly spend time communicating who recipients are and why
they are pursuing egg donation. Such information can have a powerful
influence on how women think about donation. Carla, a twenty-five-
year-old college student with a young child, detailed how her initial for-
mulation of donation as a "second job" began to change during her very
first conversation with the founder of Creative Beginnings, whom she
spoke with after seeing an advertisement in a local parenting magazine.

Rene: What made you stop and look at the ad?
Carla: Well, definitely the $5,000. That's why they put it there in bold
print. It's like, okay, I'll call. Then after finding out about the procedure, going home, talking to my husband, then it was more than just
the money. It was safety issues and stuff like that. You go through all
the pros and cons. Is it worth it? At that point, it became less of the
money and more understanding the recipient, why they're going
through all this trouble. They're spending a lot of money. Besides just
what I get, there's all the doctor bills and procedures; she has to carry
the eggs. That's what these people are going through. The only way I
could relate to that was before I had my son: we were trying to get

pregnant, so it was the anxiety, the anticipation, the peeing on the stick. I didn't have any difficulty getting pregnant, but even the one month, oh my God, I'm a day late, then it's negative, and just kind of being bummed out, remembering that feeling and sort of correlating it to what they're going through. So I gotta give it to them. I gotta help them.

Rene: So when did that change for you? How did that change from being about the money?
Carla: I think it was just [*pause*]. I talked to [the founder]. I didn't have many questions, because my mom and dad are in the medical field. But I asked her: "Besides the fact that they can't get pregnant or whatever it is, why do they have to go this far?" She explained that most recipients are women who are forty and above who don't actually produce eggs anymore. That blew me away. I had not even thought of that! After learning that, I started changing the perspective on it and putting it into more of a medical need, as opposed to just money. Don't get me wrong, I took it and spent it. But it became less of a second job and more of an I'm-helping-somebody feeling, if that makes any sense. But it was pretty soon into it, almost from the beginning. Obviously the first was the $5,000.

Pushing the focus on recipients a step further, some egg agencies allow donors to meet with them in person if both parties agree. Whereas Carla empathized with recipients because of her own efforts to become pregnant, Jane, a younger donor who did not have children, nevertheless echoed Carla in describing the shift in her "mentality" after meeting the recipients during her first cycle.

When [the founder of Creative Beginnings] found my recipient couple, I was still like, okay I got a match, and I'm going to get my money, right? And then I met the couple. They were *so* nice, and they liked me so much. After that, I felt so flattered. I didn't realize what getting a match meant, and then it was just like, wow, they want their child to look like me or to be like me, right? They were always concerned about me, always asked if I needed anything. Then after all they had given me, I mean moneywise, on the day of my egg retrieval the husband came and gave me a present. They were so appreciative, and they gave me a card. I didn't know what to do, because I'm really shy with people I don't know. I'm just like, "Oh, thank you!" I read the card later, and it said, "Thank you for helping us create our family." I was just so touched, and after that I changed my whole mentality about this is my job. I really thought I'm really helping someone and really having a great impact on someone's life.

In subsequent cycles, Jane negotiated higher fees by threatening to defect to another egg agency, but her strong interest in the money does not preclude considering donation to be "helping someone."

Jane was saving the money from egg donation to pay off student loans when she graduates. In contrast, Susan, who was divorced with a three-year-old son, needed it to cover basic living expenses. Her sister had donated at Gametes Inc. and encouraged Susan to follow in her footsteps. But Susan initially resisted, because she was worried about "messing with [my body] and not being able to have kids again." Eventually, though, she said she needed to "catch up on my bills." She explained, "I had my own house, and I didn't get any child support. Once you're a mother, you do whatever it takes, so I masked one problem with the next. We have to have electricity, and it's $100 this month, but if I pay $50, they'll keep it on. Things just built up and built up. Car insurance is due, but [my son] has got to have Christmas."

Despite her overwhelming need for the money, Susan nevertheless described receiving a gift from the recipients, whom she never met, as completely changing her mindset about paid donation.

Susan: The thing that just melted me and still does until this day—I don't know who these people were; they don't know who I am—when I went in for the retrieval, the office staff was great, and my recipients had dropped off a gift. It was a children's book. In it, she wrote a note: "You have no idea what you've done for us." At that moment, it became everything about this couple that is just so desperate to have a child that they'll do this. I'm so blessed that, honestly, I didn't even try to have a child [laughs], and these people are just destitute to have a baby. I gave the book to my child, and he wants to read it all the time. He says, "Mama, where did you get this book?" And I say, "A special friend gave this to Mommy."

Rene: They gave you this gift, and it became all about them. In your mind,
what was it about before that?
Susan: I thought about it as helping someone out, and also, I will be
completely honest, I'm a single mother, and I was significantly paid for
this. Significantly. I thought, wow, this could help us, too, you know.
But then, at that moment, it became absolutely nothing about the
money, somewhat a guilty feeling about the money. Why should they
have to pay like this to have a child?

Although most egg donation programs provide women with basic
information about the outcome of their donation (i.e., whether the recipient becomes pregnant), Gametes Inc. does not. This policy irked most of
the donors there, and Susan used gift rhetoric in saying of her recipients,
"Do I want to know when she has it? No. Do I want to know what it is?
I'd be real uneasy about that. But I do want to know that they did receive
a gift from this, that they didn't just give and give and give and not get
anything back."

Like Susan, about a third of the women reported receiving a present,
either from recipients or program staff. Valerie said that after her first
donation at Gametes Inc., the staffers gave her "a little Fabergé egg as a
gift. It's cute. The second time, they gave me a little heart." Lisa received
a postcard from OvaCorp at Christmas saying "what a great gift." But
even women who did not receive a present used the language of the gift
in describing donation, demonstrating that an actual gift exchange need
not exist for women to invoke this rhetoric.

Alongside the gift talk and gift exchange, women do receive thousands of dollars, and some egg donors deal with this seeming incongru-
ity by referencing the importance of donating for the "right reasons."
Samantha, a two-time donor who used the money to pay for school,
hopes that egg agencies "screen for someone who really cares about it,
not just they want to do it for the money. Me and the recipient, we'll
always have a small little connection, even though we never met, from
what I was able to give her physically. I just don't think [people] think of
it like that. They think of it as maybe something too medical or maybe
too impersonal." Indeed, many of the egg donors referenced similar

feelings of "caring" about recipients and sympathized with how difficult it must be to go through infertility. All but one of the women specifically said they "hoped" recipients became pregnant, compared to just a handful of the men (who tended to be those who signed on to help others).

Beth, a six-time donor who was matched for a seventh cycle, was among the most adamant about the importance of being properly motivated. In addition to working as a nanny, she was also a program assistant at OvaCorp, so she was well aware of the fees she could command. But Beth was not comfortable with "putting a price on it." She explained "I always let [the donor manager] work it out, whatever the couple can afford. I don't ask for a number, because that just doesn't seem right. It just cheapens it. It makes it seem like you're more interested in the money than actually helping the couple."

In the case of one of her recipients, Beth demonstrated just how invested she was in "helping the couple." She described how "Kate, and her husband, Frank, she wants a baby in the worst way. She's a perfect match, nationality, looks, everything. It's almost like we could be sisters." After meeting with them for the first time, Beth agreed to reduce her fee from $10,000 to $6,000 so they could afford it. "It's unheard of that you'd go down to 4,000 [dollars], but I just wanted to help her." The cycle was not successful. "Unfortunately, [Kate] didn't get pregnant, because her [uterine] lining wasn't ready." So Beth agreed to participate in an egg freezing experiment, for which she would receive $5,000, and "worked it out so Kate can get some of my eggs for free from the [experiment]. She's just a loving person. She really deserves to have a baby. They just can't afford it. It's expensive, and they're like middle-class, working, regular Joes." In interview after interview, egg donors emphasized how much they care—not about the money they were making but about the recipients they were helping.

Most significant, though, is the lack of employment rhetoric in women's discussions of donation. Even Tiffany, who was quite straightforward in discussing her strong interest in the money, still did not call donation a job. She had been matched with her first recipient, whom she was to meet the following week, but she had not yet started injections and had had limited contact with the staff at the egg agency. At this early stage in the process, she had not had much exposure to the organizational framing of egg donation as a gift, and she described money as her "number one" reason for donating. At the same time, she felt that she was "giving something to someone that they can't have for themselves." Summing up her thoughts, she concluded, "When you think about it in the long run after it's done, I think you're going to be thinking more about how much good you're doing rather than how much money you made."

Simply put, women do not believe that being paid to donate constitutes a job, and the presence of monetary exchange is not incongruous with calling donation a gift. Pam, a twenty-seven-year-old who was in nursing school and occasionally worked as a nanny, explained the distinction between paid donation and a job.

> [Egg donation] doesn't feel like a job. It's sort of like a process that you choose to undergo, and at the end, you get compensated because you've gone through all the trouble. It doesn't feel earned I guess. I didn't feel like I was working for a paycheck in this case. It almost felt like here's a little gift at the end to thank you for the trouble you've gone through. I don't know. That sounds weird to me now that I say it. I think it's because I've never put it into words before.

Several other women also discussed the importance of "choosing" to donate in distinguishing it from a job, suggesting a new instantiation of feminist pro-choice rhetoric. In making the choice to help recipients have children and in being compensated for their efforts, women articulate a conceptualization of donation that directly reflects the organizational framing of egg donation as a gift, a framing that relies heavily on gendered stereotypes of women as selfless, caring, and focused on relationships and family.

Men, in contrast, talked much less about recipients, did not report receiving thank-you notes and gifts, and did not make distinctions about donating for the right reasons. Instead, sperm donors mirror the banks' organizational framing in defining donation as a job, referencing the money, the routine deposits they must make, and the necessity of producing passable samples. Mike, who was working at several low-wage service jobs and donating two or three times a week, said,

> [Sperm donation is] just something to make some money off of now. I don't get a whole lot of money from my parents anymore, just because

they're going through a divorce and having financial trouble themselves. I'm trying to go to school to be a nurse, too. I have to study a lot, and there's not a job where I can come and make ninety bucks in half an hour. Anywhere else, I wouldn't be able to work around my school schedule. That's why I kept coming, because it's just a lot of money. I'm, like, a lifeguard, too, and I have a bunch of different other jobs. I make the most money coming here, but I treat this just like I would treat any other job.

Similarly, Kyle compared sperm donation with his other job where he works full-time. He described being a donor as "the easiest job I've ever had. I put in probably an hour a week, I don't break a sweat, I'm not doing manual labor, and I make almost as much as working forty-five hours a week loading trucks."

Paul, a college student who held part-time jobs, said that donation is not hard work but pointed to the money he receives in defining it as a "side job."

When I talk to people and make a reference to [sperm donation] as being a job, it's sort of joking. It's not really a job. I wouldn't really call it recreation [laughs]. I don't know. I guess it would be considered like maybe a little side job, because you do get paid for it. It's not really hard work or anything. It's not like you have to put in long hours in order to come here [laughs]. So it's not a job in the traditional sense of the word at all but maybe just a little side job.

In contrast to women, men reference the payment they receive in conceptualizing donation as a form of employment. Although not exactly like other kinds of work, the monetary exchange results in paid donation being categorized as a job.

Sperm donors also relied on the language of the workplace in calling the money "income" or "wages" whereas egg donors were more likely to call it a "fee" or a "price," which evokes a one-time exchange rather than steady paychecks. Women were also slightly more likely to use the term "compensation," which connotes payment for something lost, rather than "income," which connotes payment for something earned. Additionally, a fifth of the women, and none of the men, called the money a "gift." These subtle rhetorical distinctions are in keeping with the gendered organizational framing of donation, and donors are consistent with how they use such language. For example, if they described the money as "income," they did not call it a "gift" and vice versa.

Several of the men from Western Sperm Bank referred to donation as a "service," which suggests that this nonprofit organization promotes a slightly different framing of donation. Andrew, who had been a donor for the last eighteen months, noted it "is a great way to make money if you have the ability. It's also providing a service, making the world a better place for people who want to have children but for some reason aren't able to conceive." Referring to donation as a "service" can be understood as a rhetorical middle ground between gift and job. It references some elements of altruism while stopping short of calling donation a gift, and the term "providing" is more associated with masculinity, as in a breadwinner who "provides" for his family. Women almost never use this language of service provision. The one woman who called donation a "service" also called it a "gift," and none of the egg donors used the word "providing."

Andrew is unusual in mentioning recipients, who rarely appear in sperm donors' discussions of donation, primarily because bank staff do not spend much time talking about them. In fact, just one of the men knew something specific about the people who bought his sperm. Compare this to nearly 80% of the egg donors, whose knowledge of recipients ranged from knowing what state they lived in to having met them in person. Several of the men did not even have ready-made language for referring to them. Travis, who had been donating at Gametes Inc. for the last eighteen months, hesitated and said, "I don't know how to say" before calling recipients "post-injected people and their kids." Victor referred to them as "the purchasers of my samples." At some point in the interview, most of the sperm donors did make a vague reference to "helping people," but as men are not given specific information about who these people are, the way in which they help is not only abstract, but also gendered: men contribute to the lives of others through paid production, while women help particular people through compensated giving.

PROUD GIVERS VS. ALIENATED LAB RATS

These gendered conceptualizations of donation are not without consequences. In concert with organizational protocols of payment, in which women are guaranteed a negotiated sum and men are paid a flat rate for samples that pass, framing donation as a gift or a job creates systematically different experiences of being paid for parts of one's body. These effects are clear in how egg and sperm donors discussed bodily production, including the extent to which they expressed feelings of alienation from their own bodies.

Both women and men talked about the number of sex cells they generated per donation, but the rationale for their concern with bodily production differed. Men hoped to generate a high-enough sperm count to get paid, and women hoped to make enough eggs to give recipients a good chance at becoming pregnant. Mike, when asked if he could change anything about being a sperm donor, said, "I just hate sometimes when [the lab technician] tells me mine hadn't passed. Well, I did the same thing! But I just wish we could get money for every time instead of it having to pass." Travis, a salaried engineer, pointed out that sperm bank advertisements are not entirely straightforward in this regard. "It said make up to twelve hundred bucks a month. That was a little bit of a falsehood, because there's virtually no way to do that." Indeed, it would require three donations per week with all samples passing. Unlike Mike, Travis was not in "need" of the money from sperm donation, but he was still irked by the bank's practices.

Although it was not one of my interview questions, more than half the women reported how many eggs they produced per cycle. But when women raised the issue of bodily production, the focus was not on compensation. For example, Jessica, who had finished her first cycle two months before, explained,

> My eggs were kind of slow to mature, and I was kind of frustrated, not at anybody but just myself. I was like, man, I'm going to be upset if I don't give but about five or ten eggs. You just want to give as much as you can so that [the recipients will] have a chance. Finally in the end, I pulled through, and [the donor manager] said, "You're just a late bloomer." So everything worked out well. I was very happy when I woke up, and they're like "You gave seventeen," which is good. I think my friend told me the average is between ten and twenty, so it just depends. But I was glad that I gave a decent number, and it worked out well.

This sentiment, of being "frustrated" and "upset" by the prospect of not "giving" enough, is the logical outcome of a donation process that is structured as an altruistic gift exchange between participants who care about each other as well as one in which the donor will be paid regardless of bodily output.

Indeed, women were more likely to suggest that they were being paid for the *process* of donation (time, injections, surgery, and/or risk) rather than the *outcome* (eggs), and the opposite was true of men. Evincing a focus on process, Nicole, a thirty-five-year-old actress who had cycled four times, said, "Whatever thoughts I had about how much I should get as far as money and how much I shouldn't, it went right out the window, because doing those shots [*laughs*] and going to the doctor like every three days, it's a lot of time, a lot of work, a lot of recovery afterwards. So it's worth every penny." Similarly, Heather concluded that "the very fact that they offer [compensation] is kind of like they recognize that you do have to inject yourself and that you are taking risks with your life."

In contrast, men were more likely to say that they were being paid for sperm or, euphemistically, for "samples," which are the *outcome* of a donation process that involves not only masturbation, but also abstinence from sexual activity as well as eating healthy foods and getting enough sleep. For example, Fred said he decided to apply at Gametes Inc. after hearing that he could "get sixty-five bucks for samples." A similar orientation, in which the production of viable sperm is the basis for payment, is clear in Andrew's response to his mother's offer to pay him *not* to be a donor. His mother was not thrilled with the idea of having "grandchildren running around" whom she did not know, so "she sent me a check for $500. I'm like, 'All right, Mom, I won't donate for ten times then.'" At Western Sperm Bank in 2002, Andrew received $50 per passing sample.

This sort of explicit calculation demonstrates that men's conceptualizations of donation result from the sperm banks' organizational policy of conditioning payment on sperm count. For example, Manuel, a donor at Western Sperm Bank, described his routine.

> I had a routine down. I was in and out in five minutes. I'd get there, take care of business, talk to [the donor manager] for a minute or two. Overall,

the whole thing, get there and back, would take no more than half an hour. So it was worth it, because it's $50 for every usable sample. Of the twelve or thirteen [samples] in that period, I would average eight to ten [passing], so more than half in most cases. So I figure that's like, if you break it down, that's $50 for fifteen minutes of work. That's better than my job at the time.

Although Manuel mentioned the amount of time it takes to travel to and from the sperm bank, his calculations of how much this "work" is worth are based on "usable samples." Women rarely engaged in this sort of accounting, and the fact that more than half the men did suggests their orientation to donation as piecework, in which they are paid for successfully completing a particular task.

Sperm donors were also more likely than egg donors to make direct reference to donation as a commodified exchange between donor and recipient. They called recipients "customers," defined the sperm bank as the "middleman," or noted that their samples were not "on the market yet." Women did talk about the recipient's "investment" of time and money to have a child via IVF and egg donation, but they did not go so far as to refer to recipients as paying customers who purchase eggs.[11]

Ultimately, egg donors spoke with pride about the huge gift they were giving. Heather summarized her experience with egg donation at University Fertility Services.

> Giving my eggs to somebody, it's huge. Being able to look back twenty years later and just knowing that I could contribute to some lady somewhere having kids, giving that gift. The process that I had to go through wasn't a quick thing. It's something that I actually had to sit and think about, and it was a process that I had to stick through. I had to stick myself with needles. It was a big memorable event. I mean it's not like just going to see a movie or something like that. It's something I chose to do, chose to contribute to some woman somewhere.

Heather is a college student who anticipated having children one day. Erica is a Gametes Inc. donor who stays at home with her two young children. Yet in speaking of her hope that the recipients become pregnant, she revealed a similar conception of the gift, also describing it as "huge."

Erica: On some levels, I would like to know what happened, just if someone would say you got a successful pregnancy or not. But then if things didn't work out, I don't know that I would want to know. I'd almost feel like I'd be carrying that burden, even though I know it's not necessarily my fault or anything. I hate carrying around someone else's pain, but we are kind of tied to each other in this way. That might be nice, but it's also nice that we're all able to maintain our separate lives, too, because it's part of the gift.

Rene: Part of a gift in what way?
Erica: A woman is not able, for whatever reason, to have children on her own, but then you just give a couple cells, and she's able to carry on as if she could. Of course she's aware, and the child may or may not be aware, that their genetic background is different, but still she's able to carry a child, have ultrasounds, and see it move and grow and feel the kick and give birth and hold it from that first moment. That's a big thing, I know. Being able to maintain that as if it were their own. That's huge.

In contrast, men did not wax poetic about the significance of sperm donation. In fact, in response to an interview question, about a third of the sperm donors said that giving blood was a more significant form of donation. Paul, a twenty-year-old college student, noted, "There are more people that need blood. It's more a necessity, you get in a car accident or something, but nobody really needs sperm." No egg donor came to this same conclusion.[12]

Ultimately, sperm donors referenced feelings of objectification and alienation, describing their bodies as "assets" or "resources" for the sperm bank. For example, Dennis described how an encounter with staff made him think differently about "donating."

Dennis: When I had a streak of bad samples, my feeling was: whatever, they don't pay me [for those samples]; it doesn't matter. I'm donating here. What's the big deal? It'll work itself out. But they were like, "You gotta fix this now." And that took me by surprise. Oh, am I getting fired? [*laughs*] It was the first instance where I was like this is a job. They think of this as a job. You're sort of like an asset to them, and if you're not performing, they don't want to have any part of you. I finished giving my sample, and they were like, "So you've had three bad samples. I don't know what's going on. I don't know what the problem is, but you really need to fix this." I was like, "Yikes. Okay!" [*laughs*] Too much pressure there. So that was a major mindfuck. That changes the whole way I was approaching it. Now it's like you need to perform.

Rene: How had you been approaching it before?
Dennis: Just very casual. If I don't come in, whatever. If I do it, I get fifty bucks. But I wasn't thinking of it like a business, like a business commitment, like a job, which is essentially what it is really. And they purposely make it like a job, because they are running a business, and they need good samples.

Dennis donated at the feminist nonprofit Western Sperm Bank, which he nevertheless defined as a "business" where staffers make donation "like a job," which results in "pressure" placed on men to "perform."

Whereas Dennis was originally interested in donation because he was desperately in need of the money, Ben described himself as "independently wealthy" and talked about donation as an act of "charity." Yet Ben used language similar to Dennis' in outlining the spatial experience of being a sperm donor. In most of the banks, men are asked to enter and leave through a separate door from the recipients, and in each case, the "donor door" was around the side or the back of the building. As a result, Ben felt "second class" and identified himself as a "resource" that the bank needs.

Ben: You get an impression you're not really [the bank's] chief concern, that when push comes to shove, they would be trying to protect the mother more than the donor when it comes to legal issues. That's another reason why I was very careful, and I really wanted to be anonymous, because I felt when push came to shove that I'd be the one that got shoved.[13]

Rene: What gave you that impression?
Ben: Because when you go to the sperm bank, you're asked to go around the back way. When you leave, you're going back around the

back way. You're not going through the front door. I don't think it's a big deal, and I understand it. They're in business for the women. I'm just a resource they need. Their whole ideological reason is to help women empower themselves to have their own children. I understand my place in the whole scheme of things.

Later in the interview he returned to this theme and put it more bluntly. "I felt like a piece of meat almost. I felt like a cow. I'm being milked for something that I can provide." He concluded that if sperm donors were "really the chief concern, maybe they'd be paid for even the samples that weren't accepted."

Ethan echoed these feelings of alienation in his description of the difference between masturbating at home and masturbating at the sperm bank.

> What's weird about it is going into a doctor's office and jerking off. It's kind of like a sexual thing you're using in a totally nonsexual way. It's not the privacy of your own bedroom, and it's not whenever else you might choose to masturbate. This is like masturbation on demand. You're a lab rat. You can go in and smile and say all the nice things you want every morning, but they really want you for one thing. You are a walking sperm donor.

This quote is particularly striking because both Ethan and the donor manager, in independent interviews, talked about how much they liked each other. Although he had stopped donating about six months before, they were still in touch because Ethan and his wife were trying to get pregnant, and the donor manager was giving them advice about timing intercourse based on ovulation. Despite this friendship, he still described himself as "a lab rat," which demonstrates the power of the sperm banks' organizational practices to shape the experience of commodification in such a way that it induces feelings of alienation.[14]

Women, who are being paid much more money for their sex cells, did not use this same kind of harsh language. Nicole, who donated four times with four different physicians, did call one of the infertility practices a "factory" while complaining about incompetent blood draws, but this language was not directed at her own body. Indeed, she concluded the interview by talking about how egg donation had made her feel *more* "of value."

> I got on the bone marrow registry after donating [eggs]. I'm just more willing to give up my body physically to those in need. I feel like I have more of a value in some ways. It's probably part of being an actress; there's so many times that you don't get what you want, you don't get a part or whatever, and it made me feel like I wasn't of value. So this sort of makes me feel like I am of value and that there is something else for me to contribute to the world.[15]

Nicole does not mention money at all in talking about "giving up her body," and her logic directly contradicts the assumptions of commodification scholars who contend that being paid for parts of one's body is inherently dehumanizing.

CONCLUSION

In this medical market, the provision of sex cells for money is framed as a gift or a job, depending on whether the exchange occurs in an egg agency or a sperm bank. It is the prospect of financial compensation that attracts most applicants, yet egg donors respond to the organizational framing by defining paid donation as an altruistic gift that is motivated by care and concern for recipients who cannot have children. In contrast, sperm donors conceptualize paid donation as a job for which they must show up on a regular basis and produce samples with the requisite sperm count. These patterns are robust; they appear in interviews with donors at different points in their lives, with different financial situations, at different stages in the donation process, and from different donation programs in different parts of the country.

But more than just making an appearance in donors' descriptions, these organizational framings of donation have consequences. In stoking the connection between egg donor and recipient, staffers make it possible for women to construe their participation in this market as an altruistic act for which they are compensated, which seems to offer a

protective effect against other unsavory narratives that could be generated, such as being paid for body parts or even prostitution. However, at
the same time, this donor/recipient connection results in pressure on
women to engage in the emotional labor of caring about recipients, hoping they become pregnant and feeling guilty if they do not. Sperm donors
are not required to think about recipients at all, much less care about
them. But this lack of connection, combined with the fact that they are
paid based on a bodily performance that is often not up to par, results in
feelings of objectification and alienation.

There is nothing inherent in biology or technology that determines
these organizational practices. Egg agencies *could* match an individual
egg donor with multiple recipients, tell her nothing about them, and
condition payment on the number of eggs she produces. Sperm banks
could foster a one-to-one relationship between an individual sperm donor
and "his" recipient, encourage him to consider the plight of infertile
couples, and nudge recipients to send thank-you notes and presents.[16]
Men *could* be paid on the basis of process, regardless of the sperm count
in a particular deposit, as long as they produced passing samples on a
regular basis. For now, however, these exist only as counterfactual pos-
sibilities, leaving open the question of whether such changes would actually alter the experience of being paid to produce sex cells.

FIVE

Defining Connections

One potential outcome of egg and sperm donation is children, "off-spring" in the parlance of fertility programs, who are genetically related to the donors who provide the raw materials of conception. Scholars and the public alike have been fascinated by the kinship permutations made possible by reproductive technologies, which can result in the splitting of motherhood and fatherhood into genetic, gestational, and social components. In other words, as many as three individuals might contribute biologically to the birth of a single child: the woman who provides the egg, the man who provides the sperm, and the woman who carries the pregnancy to term. These roles may or may not overlap with those of the social parents, the people who care for the child once it is born.

Most social science research on assisted reproduction focuses on recipients, the "intended parents," and examines how different sorts of biological and social connections shape the relationships they develop with their children. More recently, the children themselves, many of whom are now adults, have become more vocal about their experiences as donor-conceived children.[1] (Although, in many cases, parents who use donated gametes do not tell their children, keeping their genetic origins a secret.[2]) For example, the Donor Sibling Registry is a website founded in 2000 by a woman who used donated sperm to conceive her son. She was frustrated by the sperm bank's insistence on anonymity, and she wanted to create a place where donors and offspring who wanted to could find each other. The site now has more than 25,000 members, including egg and sperm donors, recipient parents, and "donor-conceived people." It has also provided an opportunity for half-siblings to meet each other, and some "family reunions," involving ten or fifteen children who are all related to one another through the same donor, have appeared on television news magazines such as *60 Minutes*.

Despite the increasing attention to issues of kinship, there is still very little known about how *donors* understand their position in these brave new families.[3] To what extent do egg and sperm donors feel a connection to the children born of their donations, and how do they define that connection? Generally speaking, there is a societal expectation that women donating eggs will feel more of a connection than men donating sperm. This expectation is driven by a cultural belief in "maternal instinct," which forms from an amalgam of biological and cultural assumptions about women and their bodies. One influential version of this belief derives from evolutionary psychology. It contends that women have fewer eggs than men have sperm, that it takes more biological effort to produce eggs and bear children, and thus women are more "invested" in offspring than men are.

This is certainly the view of some of the most prominent fertility doctors in the country. When I asked a past president of ASRM what he thinks of as "open questions" in gamete donation, he said it is important to know more about "what happens on the other side of the door. What happens to the donors? Do they forget it, or is it part of their life for the rest of their lives?" He went on to speculate:

Physician: I would suspect that this is very different in women than in men. The sperm donors probably couldn't give a hoot about what happened to those kids. They did it for the money. It was easy to collect the sperm and [then] good-bye. The women, I think, will have an investment.

Rene: Where does that investment come from?
Physician: Because women have children. Women relate very differently to children than men.

In this view, biology is at the root of gender differences in how egg and sperm donors relate to offspring: female bodies bear babies and thus women are more invested in children.

Social scientists challenge the idea of maternal instinct as overly reliant on a deterministic view of biology. Just as with biological sex differences, biological ties in the realm of kinship can be differently understood depending on the social context in which they are being referenced. Marilyn Strathern initially raised this point in the context of reproductive technologies, suggesting that they might change the ways in which biology is mobilized in defining relatedness. The studies that followed have demonstrated just how malleable the meaning of biological ties can be.[4] Depending on which element—genetics or gestation—is being provided by someone other than the intended parents, that particular element is downplayed. For example, a surrogate mother who carries a fetus conceived from the egg and sperm of the intended parents will downplay her gestational connection in favor of highlighting the female recipient's genetic connection to the child, defining her as the "real mother."[5] In another example, an infertile woman who uses donated eggs to conceive a fetus that she herself will carry is likely to downplay the egg donor's genetic connection in favor of highlighting her own gestational role.

As egg and sperm donors, women and men make parallel contributions to reproduction: each provides cells filled with genetic material, but they will not carry the pregnancy or care for the child once it is born. This raises the question of whether egg and sperm donors understand this genetic contribution in the same way. In fact, they do not. In direct contrast to notions of maternal instinct, egg donors insist that they are *not* mothers to children born of their eggs, but sperm donors have a straightforward view of themselves as fathers.

In this chapter, I examine how it is that donors come to these conclusions and look closely at how women and men define their connection to offspring, including the extent to which they make distinctions between biological and social parenthood. I point to the ways that donors' views are influenced by organizational practices, namely the emphasis on the donor/recipient relationship in egg agencies and the lack thereof in sperm banks. I conclude with a discussion of how donors' perceptions reflect broader cultural norms around procreation, particularly the longstanding tradition in Western culture that identifies the male role in reproduction as primary.

"I'M A FATHER!"

Most sperm donors define themselves as fathers to children born of their donations.[6] Such definitions appeared throughout my interviews and ranged from flippant quips to more serious and subtle discussions of the dimensions of this paternal relationship. The flippant references were more likely to come from younger donors, such as Paul, a twenty-year-old college student who described one of his considerations in deciding to become a donor. "It was like a week and a half or two trying to think everything over, whether or not I actually wanted to have children that I didn't know about [laughs]." Referencing their participation in the banks' identity-release programs (in which donors agree to future contact with offspring), several men echoed Isaac, a twenty-two-year-old student who noted that one day there could be someone who "shows up on my doorstep saying, 'Hey, Pops, how you doing?'" Mike, a twenty-two-year-old virgin, joked, "I have more kids without having sex than any of [my friends] will actually doing it." Walt, a nineteen-year-old firefighter, explained how in the four months since he began donating, he started to think not just about the money he was making but about the "kids that you could have later. Like if you're sitting there at the bar when you're forty and start hitting on an eighteen-year-old girl, it could be your daughter [laughs]."

Older sperm donors also defined themselves as fathers, but their understanding of this role reflects the changing life experiences of men in their thirties and forties. For example, a few months after our interview, Ethan, a thirty-nine-year-old graduate student, found out his wife was expecting their first child. He contacted me to say that, as a result, some of his views about being a donor had changed, and he agreed to a follow-up interview. He is the only donor I interviewed twice. Ethan described his thoughts after his wife's positive pregnancy test.

> A lot of stuff goes through your mind the next few days. One of them was, "Oh yeah, there's other children out there. Maybe that was a mistake, that identity-release." I can't remember exactly what felt funny, but it just felt funny for a moment where it never felt funny before. Before it felt fun and interesting that I might meet these children some day. But this, all of a sudden now, when you have your own children, when you've got your own family and world going on here, that seemed like such an extraneous thing that I did that shouldn't come back and involve itself in your family.

He described this as his initial reaction, but after a little bit of time passed, he spoke with the donor manager at Western Sperm Bank and "came back down to earth. It's all good. [The donor manager] explained to me some of the neat things. The kids were sending pictures, and they're starting now to meet their parents." In the first quote, Ethan distinguishes the offspring, the "other children," from his "own children" and his "own family," but in the second quote, he still refers to sperm donors as "parents" to "kids" who are born from donation.

Another example of this shifting orientation toward offspring comes from Joe, who was in his late forties at the time of our interview. Fifteen years earlier, he had signed on to donate after being encouraged by his girlfriend, because neither was particularly interested in having children. As an engineer, he had no need for the money from donation, and, in fact, he estimated spending more on fast food in a month than he earned at the sperm bank. Years later, after the relationship and the donations had ended, he married a different woman, and they tried to have a child together. "When it turned out the odds were probably not going to be in our favor, there was some resentment. I had done this [sperm donation], and she was not able to get pregnant."

As an identity-release donor, Joe expressed concern about how his wife would react if the people he referred to as "offspring" contacted him in the future. This is a distinct possibility, because he has learned that several recipients have had children. "I was actually surprised at my feelings when I found out the first birth had occurred, stronger feelings than I expected, somewhat pride, somewhat joy, probably a smaller subset of what an actual father feels when he and a partner have a kid." Although Joe distinguished his contribution as a sperm donor from that of an "actual father," he was curious to meet the offspring, explaining, "I have siblings, nieces, nephews, and so on. There's always a question of which traits are inherited and which are learned, nature versus nurture, so it would be very interesting to see which traits you recognize." In fact, his curiosity was quite strong: he had considered moving to a different country to work or retire but put these plans off in part to be more available to meet with offspring who would be turning eighteen in the next few years. At the same time, he said, "There's also a definite limitation on my part as to how much of a relationship. I have my life. I am definitely interested, but I am also married."

Although several of the older donors had contemplated some sort of meeting in the future, Nathan was the only man I interviewed who had actually met children born from his donations. In what the Gametes Inc. staff said was an extremely unusual turn of events, Nathan agreed to be in touch with several different recipients when their children were still quite young. At the beginning of the correspondence, all letters went through bank staffers, who excised any identifying information, but Nathan grew impatient with this arrangement and asked if he could just e-mail directly with the recipients. E-mails led to phone calls that led to conversations via webcam and then, the weekend before our interview, to a "family" reunion on a beach a few hours away. Nathan joined two families, both headed by lesbian couples, who had conceived children with his sperm and were vacationing together. He recalled his initial conversations with the children: "When we meet up, 'You're my dad?' 'Yes, I am.' 'I'm your son?' 'Yes, you are.' 'Well, let's go play.' And off we go. It's like nothing to them. It's readily accepted."

Like most other donors, Nathan was originally interested in the money he could earn from donation. That was fifteen years ago. "I was in school, going to work, and I heard this advertisement on the radio on how to make extra money. Great, no problem. Make extra money by just tossing off. Fantastic! So there was no real thought of children or off-spring down the line or consequences or benefits at all, from any of it. It was just a go-in-and-do-what-you're-normally-going-to-do-at-night and get paid [*laughs*]." Within five or six years, however, he faced a "turning point" about whether he wanted to continue donating sperm: "I don't plan on getting married. I have no aspirations to get married. I have no children of my own, and I'm not going to raise children by myself. So, the question was, do you really want to keep doing this? Do you want to have more children out there? Why not? I mean, it's a great thing. So, I just kept on going. They still gave you money, but the money was no longer a deciding factor."

At thirty-eight, Nathan was unmarried and still working odd jobs. Although he would like to have children of his own, he did not want to do it by himself, nor did he feel financially prepared. "It wouldn't be fair to the kids, because I couldn't give them everything they need, not right now." So as recipients were in and out of touch as their own lives changed, Nathan looked forward to meeting more offspring. "It kills me to know that there are more out there that I'll probably never meet, because I want to see them when they grow up, how they progress, and how they change through life, if they go through the same things and handle the same things that I did, the same way I did."

At the same time, he was very aware that his presence in the children's lives is at the discretion of their parents. In summing up his experiences as a sperm donor, he said,

Getting letters and pictures, you're elated. You're happy. You got this new sense of being, this new purpose, but it's just out of reach. You can't do anything with it. I got kids. That's great. I can go make more, but that's as far as it goes. Fuck [*laughs*]. It kind of leaves you hanging, wanting more. You want the parents to be calling you right then and there going, "Hey little Nathan, [*imitates a baby crying*] that's your kid." You want to be a part of it, but you know you can't, not unless they invite you into that world. And you have to be really careful once you're in. You can't step on toes and whatnot. And that brings it up to this point, where I'm actually being kind of rolled into the fold. It's like being rolled into a wave. You know where you are, you know your situation, but you're not exactly sure how to kick yourself up left or right. It's all new.

Nathan was very unusual among sperm donors in that he had met the children and placed so much emphasis on his relationship with them, but he was not at all unusual in calling himself a father to these children, in considering the children to be "his." Although the conceptualization of this paternal role may change alongside a donor's changing life circumstances, younger men and older men, those who have children of their own and those who do not, are fairly uniform in identifying themselves as fathers to children conceived with their sperm.

"JUST AN EGG"

Most egg donors, who have exactly the same genetic relationship to offspring as sperm donors, come to the opposite conclusion: they are *not* mothers.[7] In interview after interview, women used similar phrasing to define their contribution as "just an egg." Tiffany, a twenty-five-year-old divorcée who had no children of her own, was in the earliest stages of donating. She was matched to recipients she was meeting the following week, but she had not yet begun injecting fertility medications. Here, she relies on a comparison between eggs and blood in explaining why she felt no "attachment whatsoever."

> There is one friend that does not like the fact that I'm doing [egg donation]. She said, "I don't see how you can do that. There's going to be a little Tiffany running around."[8] And I don't consider it that way. I mean, I donate my blood. I don't consider my blood being out there in any way. I don't feel an attachment whatsoever. It's not like I carried the kid. If I carried the kid, I could see an attachment, and I would consider it a little me running around. But just because it's my egg, I don't consider it me. I mean, it is a part of you, but you don't have a bond with it. Like if you scrape yourself and you lose some blood, you're not thinking twice: clean that up. You don't think, "Oh my God, I'm leaking! That's part of me. Get it all up, and save it." So that's the same way I feel about the eggs. You don't have a bond. You don't want to save it. It hasn't developed into anything to love at that point.

The same age as Tiffany, Carla was married with a young child. She was going to school and working as a waitress in a cocktail bar when she saw an ad offering $5,000 to become an egg donor. She had finished her first cycle about a year before our interview. Although she believed that "having kids is big and would wish that for anybody," she identified the offspring as the *recipient's* child, pointing to the importance of "giving" in explaining why she felt "no connection."

Carla: When it actually comes out of my body, it's just a little seed. This whole thing nine months later, I make no connection with that to me. That's their child, and thank God they had that child.

Rene: How does it go from this little seed that comes from you to their child?
Carla: I don't know. I think it's just giving. I think if I went out and painted somebody's house, I put all the sweat and had the pride of doing that, but then they live in it. It has nothing to do with me. That's their house, and I'm so glad that they have a nice painted house. But I'm not going to drive by every day and say, "Ooh, I painted that house." After that, it has nothing to do with me. I have the satisfaction of knowing that somebody is happy, and that's it.

There is a seeming contradiction between egg donors who describe what they are giving as a "huge" gift and then say in the very next breath that it is "just an egg." Yet Carla's quote makes clear that it is the possibility of a child that makes egg donation "huge" while what it is that egg donors give—"a little seed" or "a couple of cells"—is small.

It follows logically that women who do not feel attached to their eggs as long as they are gestated in another woman's body would find the prospect of surrogacy daunting. In fact, nearly three-quarters of the egg donors mentioned surrogacy at some point in the interview, with most echoing Kim in stating their absolute unwillingness to even consider the possibility.

I think I would be too emotionally attached. I cannot imagine somebody growing inside of me and not keeping it. I would never consider being a surrogate. Ever. Not even for a brother or sister. I love them to death, but I don't think I could do that. Being an egg donor, it's not a tangible thing. It's not in me. I mean, it came out of me, but it's just like giving blood. You're giving something away, and you don't see it again. It goes into somebody else's body. It's gone.

Rosa, a thirty-two-year-old mother of four, was the only egg donor I interviewed who had also been a surrogate mother. As a gestational surrogate, she did not provide the eggs and thus had no genetic connection to the fetus she carried. Here, she describes the path she took from blood donor to egg donor to surrogate.

Before anything else, the first thing I did was donate blood. You hope you get a good nurse that will get your vein the first time. You go in with the expectation of coming in and out right away, and then I get that Girl Scout kind of feeling in the end, like hey, I feel good about myself. The egg donation is really, really different, because it's more personal. It's a bigger thing. It's more directive of a uniqueness. You're going to do something specifically for an egg for somebody else to carry. It's not like the blood; you don't know where it's going to go. You have your blood in somebody else, and they go on with their life, but you're not creating a life. You're just maybe prolonging a life. [In egg donation] you're making that one connection that hopefully will cling on and that life will evolve. It will create somebody. With blood, I didn't think I was ever going to do egg donation. It kind of goes into steps, and then the biggest step to me was the surrogacy. So it's just like boom, boom, boom!

Rosa donated eggs through OvaCorp, which is part of a company that includes a surrogacy agency. After Rosa's two egg donation cycles, the donor manager at OvaCorp called to ask if she would consider becoming a surrogate mother. She thought it over, discussed it with her husband, and decided to meet the prospective recipient couple. As an egg donor, she had not met the recipients, and she contrasts that experience with surrogacy.

[In egg donation,] you have a little cramping afterwards, and then okay, hey, well, that's it. It's less involved. You just went in for that reason to help somebody out, and that's it. With the surrogacy, it was so different because of the process. You meet them. You get to know them. You go out with them. You e-mail them. For nine months, maybe a year, your life revolves around them, so you make sure to let them know you're doing fine. Because if I'm doing fine, then the baby is doing fine. Have you eaten, did you rest, did you sleep, are you okay? And of course, I'm just waddling. I was like this big old mama. It's just a big experience.

Like many of the egg donors, Rosa distinguishes the eggs that go out-side of her body to become part of someone else's child from carrying inside her body a child to whom she has no genetic connection. At no point did she define herself as a mother to either of these children.

For the last several months of the surrogate pregnancy, Rosa was on bed rest because she was pregnant with twins. During a routine checkup, the clinicians found that one of the fetuses was in distress and ordered an emergency C-section. The recipient couple lived overseas and could not get there in time for the birth, so one of the psychologists from the surrogacy agency was in the delivery room taking pictures. Rosa ex-plained what happened.

> We thought everything was going to be great, but the one that had all that stress had Trisomy 18. She was not even going to be compatible [with life]; we just knew it from then on. She lived for three days, and on the 16th, we had to let her go. I didn't want her to go alone, so out of, I don't know what it was. It was like a calling for me to be there for the baby. They had to unplug her. I told [the psychologist], "I want to be there; the parents are not here yet. They can't just let her go. She needs some kind of dignity to leave this world." So I held her, and they gave me the little quilt to hold her in. She was so cute, just like a little doll, so tiny. [The psychologist] told me I didn't have to do that. It's not part of the contract. There she goes with all the papers. I said, "You know what? This is just, it's my duty to do it, be-cause I carried this child. I want to be there to say good-bye to her." It was one of the hardest things I ever did. I'd never seen something like that in my life, to let go of a child like that, to just let it go. I just cried and cried.

Rosa continued to stay in touch with the recipients, and the first time they saw each other after the birth was during a layover on their next trip to the United States. Their surviving daughter had just had her first birthday, and when I asked how it was to see her again, Rosa said, "I wanted to hug her! [*laughs*] I was just like, 'Oh my God, I finally get to hold her again.' The last time I held her was when she was newborn. She was already trying to walk, and my reaction is just like wow, so fast, she's already walking. It just grabs you. It just tugs at your heart to know that that little child was in me and to know that they finally have a child. It's just, it's a good feeling."

As an egg donor, Rosa downplayed her genetic connection and empha-sized the recipient's gestational connection, noting the importance of being able to carry the pregnancy and give birth. As a surrogate, she downplayed her own gestational connection in favor of emphasizing the recipient's genetic connection, identifying the little girl as "their child."[9] Even in her description of the traumatic birth scene, the recipients are "the parents." Indeed, the only time Rosa used familial language to describe her relationships in this realm was in reference to the surrogacy recipient, with whom she felt "kind of like a kinship, because I guess she's always going to see me as a person that helped her have a child, and I'm always going to see her like the lady that I helped, so it's reciprocal."

INFORMATION, IDENTITY-RELEASE, AND THE FUTURE

Given that egg and sperm donors define their relationship to offspring in such different ways, with men identifying themselves as fathers but women not considering themselves mothers, it is surprising to find that they express similar feelings about potentially meeting the children at some point in the future. Nearly all of the donors discussed this possi-bility, and egg and sperm donors alike were willing to meet with those who requested it.

For some women and men, the prospect of offspring is quite concrete, yet others have no idea whether children have been born. This is be-cause egg agencies and sperm banks vary in the extent to which they share information about offspring with donors. On the West Coast, staffers at the two sperm banks generally provided details only if the men asked, while staffers at the two egg agencies were more proactive, checking in with women about whether they wanted to know the out-come of their donations. Indeed, all of the egg donors at Creative Begin-nings and OvaCorp knew whether recipients had become pregnant or given birth, but just two-thirds of the men at Western Sperm Bank did.[10] For example, Manuel, who began donating nearly two years ago, ex-plained, "I don't know how many people or kids or what. They don't tell us anything, other than 'You're doing a good job. Keep up the good work.' They don't really give us too much information."

On the East Coast, Gametes Inc. maintains different policies for egg and sperm donors. The sperm bank began offering identity-release as an option in 2001, and like their counterparts on the West Coast, staffers readily share information with sperm donors who inquire. However, just 25% of the men who had been donating long enough for their samples to be listed for sale had any information about recipients purchasing their samples, becoming pregnant, or giving birth. In a surprising contrast, Gametes Inc. does not offer an identity-release option for women, which is true of most egg agencies but striking in a company that sells both eggs and sperm. Moreover, Gametes Inc.'s egg agency staff members, who work just down the hall from the sperm bank staff, refuse to provide any information whatsoever to women about what happens with their donations. All but one of the egg donors expressed chagrin at this policy though generally they were more interested in knowing whether the recipient became pregnant than in learning any details about the children.

Those egg and sperm donors who did have information about outcomes reported that their recipients had become pregnant or given birth anywhere from zero to four times.[11] Several of the sperm donors who said they finally decided to ask about offspring expressed surprise at how few births there had been. In fact, reproductive technologies have relatively low success rates, so it might be the case that donors who are not given concrete information are more likely to assume that their donations result in children.[12]

Regardless of whether they knew that offspring actually existed, egg and sperm donors spoke about the possibility of meeting them in the future, and most exhibited a mild curiosity in seeing how the children "turn out." Indeed, about half the donors referenced an imagined future for the children, and these ranged from images of delinquent teenagers who start fires to ideas that the offspring could be lawyers, doctors, or even president of the United States. Ben, a twenty-six-year-old who considered donating his genes to be a charitable act, described the person he hoped to encounter eighteen years from now. "I don't want to know that, 'Hey Dad, I just got out of jail [laughs], just wanted to see how things were going, because my parents threw me out.' That's not something I want to see. I want to see, 'Hey Dad, I just made Harvard, and I just wanted you to know before I went. Everything's cool, and I appreciate you going out of your way those years back to make me.' "

More than just mild curiosity, which often revolves around what the child looks like, a substantial minority of donors—about 40% of the women and men I interviewed—conveyed feeling some sense of responsibility to offspring. Here, Carla, who was twenty-five and married with a young child, thinks through the ramifications of a future meeting.

Carla: If they ever grow up and decided they wanted to come meet me, I would be open to it. I'd really feel like I'd have to have some discussion with their parents first and find out if there are issues behind this. Is there some family drama going on that is making this child seek me out, because I'm not, I was just the seed [*laughs*]. I would definitely be supportive of this person, not as my child, but this is a person that, if I can help, I will. So yeah, if I ever was contacted, I think it would have to be from the parents. If the child just came knocking on my door one day, I would say, "I don't know who you are," and then I would call her parents. "Okay, you can come in." Any questions, I would answer everything I could. If they said, "I want to have a relationship with you," it would be—I don't know if I could do that, because they have the wrong idea. They're searching for something else, because their parents are at home. And that could very well happen, and we just deal with it I guess, find out how it goes [*laughs*]. I don't think I would ever seek them out, because, I mean, it's not mine. And I don't mean that rudely, but it's not. Every now and then, you have that urge. Maybe if I knew where the child was going to school, maybe I'd just drive by and see what they look like. I wouldn't mind being sent one picture, just for the physical part of it. How much did I put into this? It's just to have, I don't know, not have to question what they look like. That's a big thing.

Rene: How is it a big thing?
Carla: [*pause*] I don't know if it's pride or what [*laughs*]. Did you get my nose? But I think that would be the only thing. I'd hope that the child's happy, and then I'd hope that the child is beautiful.

As Carla does, most egg and sperm donors define the sense of responsibility in terms of providing information, either medical history or family background. However, a few of the donors did go so far as to say they would probably try to help if the child needed financial assistance or a place to live.

For sperm donors, the idea that they might meet offspring at some point in the future is clearly tied to their participation in the banks' identity-release programs. Greg, a young college student who donated at Gametes Inc., described his interest in such a meeting.

Greg: My understanding is that twenty years from now, when the woman has her baby and her baby is older, then either she or the kid can contact me for the sole purpose of saying, "All right, well, now you're forty, now you're fifty, is there any kind of medical problems that have developed that I should be aware of?" I thought that was okay, because I have no legal responsibilities to the kid, and it's at my own discretion whether or not I kind of want to know the kid. I may want to meet him[13] just to see how it turned out [*laughs*], but I don't think I'd ever get attached to them or anything like that.

Rene: To see how they turn out in what way?
Greg: Just kind of this is one possibility of how my genes could have turned out. Being a [science] major, I look at everything in probabilities and statistics and all the different ways things work out. So I guess if the kid ever called me, I'd kind of want to meet him, just to say this is one possible outcome of me having children. And then after that, I would probably just put it in the back of my head and move on.

Carla and Greg are similar in that they are both willing to meet offspring in the future, but Carla downplays her role by consistently calling the recipients "parents" and Greg underscores his own contribution by privileging the importance of his genes in how the child "turns out."

Gametes Inc. pays 50% more per sample to identity-release donors than it does to anonymous donors. Western Sperm Bank does not offer additional compensation to identity-release donors, so this is probably why just about half the men with posted profiles there are identity-release, compared to about two-thirds of the men at Gametes Inc.[14] Indeed, several of the Gametes Inc. donors described it as a hefty financial incentive. Walt, a nineteen-year-old who was donating to make extra money, responded to my question about what influenced his decision to be identity-release by stating bluntly, "The money." When I asked if it was a difficult decision, he said, "Not really, because I really don't mind if they look me up or not." Kyle, a twenty-two-year-old student, agreed that the decision was "not too difficult."

> I'd say on a [scale from] one to ten, with ten being the hardest, it was probably about a five or six. It wasn't super hard. I thought the money is kind of like a weight on a scale, the difference between $65 and $100 [per sample]. When you think about a whole week, I come Monday, Wednesday, Friday. I'm more a day-to-day person, and I'm thinking long term, eighteen years from now, they would be able to call me. But if I don't sell good, if you don't get out enough information, somebody might be kind of hesitant to buy your specimens. If you can't give them what they want to know, they won't buy it, and then I wouldn't be able to come in. [The sperm bank] might say 'We've got enough stock.' For me to maintain my lifestyle, I need a steady paycheck coming in just like my other job.

In contrast, when Western Sperm Bank donors explained their reasons for participating in the identity-release program, they were more likely to reference the offspring's welfare. Andrew, who like Walt and Kyle, signed on to donate for the extra money, said,

> I am [identity] release, but that's more toward the children's benefit than anything for me. I can understand how if you were a product of a sperm donation, you might be curious as to what the other donor of whatever genetic material you have is like, what their personality is like, their likes and dislikes, that type of thing. I can understand how there'd be curiosity, and not knowing where you come from would be a question that children might have. That's why I agreed to do it.

More and more sperm banks are creating an identity-release option to attract recipient clients.[15] However, when banks provide monetary incentives for donors to sign on, it is likely to focus men's attention on short-term gains rather than long-term ramifications. As a result, it remains to be seen whether those donors who are paid to participate will be as committed to staying in touch with the bank and following through on their commitment to be in contact with offspring at least two decades into the future.

SPERM : FATHER :: EGG : NOT-MOTHER

To return to the finding that sperm donors think of themselves as fathers and egg donors consider themselves not-mothers, the question remains: why does this difference exist, especially given that both women and men are making parallel contributions to reproduction? Looking more closely at how donors discuss their connections to offspring reveals an explanation that relies on a distinction between biological and social parenthood (distinguishing between the person who provides the genetic material or gestates the fetus and the person who raises the child). Nearly all of the egg donors made such a distinction, but just about half of the sperm donors did.

When men do differentiate between the person providing sperm and the person providing care, they do so not to say that they are not fathers but that they are a particular kind of father. Dennis, a twenty-four-year-old with no children of his own, explained,

> The father's the person who's there, the one who's doing the work, and I absolutely believe that environment greatly affects how a person turns out, no matter what kind of genes they have. So the only way to be a true father is to have a child and raise it, and there's no way of doing that as a donor. And yet I'm really intrigued by the idea that someone may turn eighteen and be like, "I know that I was donated sperm, and I'm curious to find out who my father was," actually encountering the person who's like, "Hey, I am the result of your genetic system." I think it'd be great to see how someone turned out. What environment, how did they grow up? What was their family like? How did they deal with being a child of a donor? I would love to have that experience, which is why I'm an identity-release person.

Dennis notes the role of nurture before returning to a more deterministic view of nature. The child is "donated sperm," and there is no mention of the recipient's "genetic system" as playing a part. The rearing family provides an "environment," but at base, the offspring is still the "child of a donor." Later in the interview, Dennis employed kinship language in defining his connection to the child.

Even though I may never meet this kid or I may run into them on the street and never know it, but just the fact that there is that sort of connection. It's also sort of a fatalism thing. Figure get it out there [*laughs*], as crude as that sounds, because if something were to happen to me tomorrow, I might still have a kid out there who's a Baby [Dennis' last name]. Their name may not be the same, but they're going to be a part of my dad, a part of my grandfather, a part of my mom. It's going to be a part of the family, and I think it's a damn good family.

When women distinguish biological and social parenthood, they do so in the service of defining themselves as not-mothers. There are two aspects of this definition, both of which appear in each of the following quotes. First, egg donors routinely break out reproduction into multiple stages, differentiating conception, pregnancy, birth, and caregiving. Second, as a result of the emphasis on recipients in egg agencies, women evinced more awareness of the people to whom they were donating than did men. In fact, nearly 70% of the women pointed out that their eggs would go into another woman's body, a detail noted by just 5% of the sperm donors.

Susan, a twenty-four-year-old with a young son, had donated twice through Gametes Inc. She described the offspring from her donation.

This is not my baby, because she [the recipient] nourishes this baby for nine months. There's an egg and there's a sperm, which create a child, but everything that goes into her body is put into this child's body. She's making everything to do with this child. This baby is not mine.

Olivia, a four-time donor at Creative Beginnings, was about the same age as Susan but had no children. She explained how her friends reacted to her decision to become a donor.

My friends thought I was crazy. They were like, "What are you doing? Technically, if a baby is born, that's your baby." And I just thought, "No." I mean, it might have my physical characteristics, or it might have my genetics, but I'm not the one bearing that child. I'm not the one going to the hospital every couple of weeks to make sure the pregnancy is going well. I'm not the one that's going to be there when the child is born. I'm not the one taking care of the child once it is born.

Erica, a twenty-seven-year-old two-time donor at Gametes Inc., references her experience as a mother of two young children in explaining why she is not the mother to offspring from her donation.

As a mother, I can't imagine carrying a child and giving birth to it and holding it and then giving it to someone else. Even though the eggs obviously carry a ton of genetic information, it's still just an egg. There's no heart, no brain. It's not like it's anything you bonded with or chose not to bond with.

Megan, a twenty-two-year-old who plans to have children in the future, had recently donated for the first time through Creative Beginnings. She responded to a question about the difference between the offspring and the children she plans to have someday.

The difference between me being a mother one day and realistically already having offspring in the world is going to be a big difference, because I will have no influence whatsoever on that offspring. That's really a complicated question. From day one, I am responsible, me and my future husband, who doesn't exist right now [*laughs*]. We will together be responsible for a child. I feel like my influence is what's going to be the big part of making an offspring from my own body mine, whereas I can donate, and there could be an offspring of my genetic makeup out there, but it's not mine, because I've had no part in its being raised or even in its conception. I mean the conception happened, and I wasn't there for it [*laughs*], and that's a big part of it. If I'm not there for any of the growth process, I feel like there's no tie there. Whatever person this baby becomes, it'll all depend on what its parents were like, not necessarily on genetic makeup. But my own child, I would be there for everything. I don't have that sense of mine when it comes to the baby that they will be having. I don't feel a connection.

Not only do women point to more stages in reproduction, they are also more likely to refer to each stage as contingent, as possible but not inevitable. Egg donors are more likely than sperm donors to specify their donation as eggs, which are mixed with sperm, which *might* result in the creation of embryos, which *might* implant in another woman's uterus, which *might* result in a successful pregnancy, which *might* result in the birth of a child.[16] For egg donors, then, reproduction looks like this:

     ?   ?   ?

Eggs → Fertilization → Implantation → Pregnancy → Birth → Child rearing

Men, who hear less about recipients, draw a more direct line from sperm to baby and assign much less uncertainty to the process. For sperm donors, reproduction looks like this:

Sperm → Baby

In part, these views, which are held by donors at different stages in life and living in different parts of the country, are shaped by donation program protocols. At egg agencies and sperm banks, staffers draw on cultural norms of maternal femininity and paternal masculinity to recruit and market donors, but they do not actually want donors to see themselves as mothers and fathers. (This could lead to complicated and messy battles over custody, which has occasionally occurred in the realm of surrogate motherhood.) But it remains a distinct possibility, given that women and men are providing genetic material in a society that defines biological ties as significant and familial.[17]

So while the last thing most donors would want is to be responsible for offspring, staffers take precautions to ensure that this does not happen, from requiring donors to sign contracts giving up all parental rights to insisting that all parties to the donation remain relatively anonymous. For example, sperm banks require that offspring be at least eighteen before receiving identifying information about the donor. Egg agency staffers are less adamant about anonymity, but they spend a lot of time coaching women about how to conceptualize their relationship to offspring, insisting that women are "just" providing eggs, not becoming mothers. Beth, a six-time donor who now works at OvaCorp, called it a "main focus. [The agency] and the psychologist really want to make sure you understand what happens afterwards, that you understand that this is not your child, that you know what you're getting into, and that it won't really bother you years later. It's an egg, and you drop an egg every month with your menstrual cycle."

In looking at the underlying causes of the donors' views and the staffs' protocols, it appears that both are referencing age-old beliefs about the role of men and women in procreation. From the time of the ancient Greeks, there has been a long tradition of identifying the male contribution as primary, a view of reproduction in which men provide the generative seed and women provide the nurturing soil.[18] Noting this distinction, anthropologist Carol Delaney makes the argument that maternity and paternity are not purely physical relationships. Instead, she believes they are "concepts" that cannot be abstracted from the cultural systems in which they are made meaningful. She writes that in the West,

> Paternity is not the semantic equivalent of maternity. Traditionally, even the physiological contribution to the child was coded differently for men and women, and therefore their connexion to the child was imagined as different. Maternity has meant giving nurture and giving birth. Paternity has meant the primary, essential, and creative role.[19]

Sperm donors who draw a short line from sperm to baby and sperm banks that institutionalize identity-release programs are referencing just this view of paternity, pointing to the man's contribution as crucial in shaping who the child becomes. Likewise, egg donors and egg agencies mobilize this view of maternity, de-emphasizing the importance of the egg in favor of highlighting the gestational or caregiving components and pointing to the recipient as the "real" mother, the one who nurtures.

One corollary to the view that fathers are creators and mothers are nurturers is that men who do not nurture are still fathers, yet women who do not nurture are censured as bad mothers. Emotionally distant fathers, absent fathers, and other "deadbeat dads" may not be held in the highest regard, but they are still fathers. In contrast, there is enormous cultural pressure on women to practice what Sharon Hays calls "intensive mothering." Those women who do not nurture their children, and particularly those who are distant or absent, violate the cultural expectation of maternal instinct and are considered nothing less than unnatural.[20] For this reason, egg agencies and egg donors both have a powerful incentive to define egg donors as not-mothers. If egg donors were categorized as mothers, then, culturally speaking, they would be the worst kind of mothers. Not only are they not nurturing their children, they are selling them for $5,000 and never looking back.

CONCLUSION

It turns out that the former president of ASRM quoted at the beginning of this chapter was right: egg and sperm donors have very different understandings of their relationship to offspring but not quite in the way he expected. Men do "give a hoot," considering the provision of sperm to be essential in defining who is a father. Women, who do not show any signs of slavishly responding to some internal maternal instinct, believe that there are too many intervening stages between the eggs they provide and the babies that result to consider themselves mothers.

These conceptualizations are buttressed by organizational practices. The gift rhetoric in egg agencies serves to highlight the importance of what the egg donor is doing for the *recipient*, making it possible for *her* to have a child and become a mother. In contrast, the identity-release programs in sperm banks work to underscore the significance of the *donor's* genetic contribution, making it difficult for men to *not* think of themselves as integral in the lives of offspring.

Egg and sperm donors' orientations to offspring are also profoundly shaped by cultural depictions of motherhood and fatherhood in twenty-first-century America, depictions with deep roots in Western philosophical and medical traditions that are given a modern spin in the realm of assisted reproduction. The elements of maternity are separable, which makes it possible to associate (or not associate) genetics, gestation, and caregiving with motherhood. In contrast, the elements of paternity are not so easily partitioned; the sperm provider is still a father of some sort.

Indeed, this study reveals that the distinction between biological and social parenthood is gendered. Women and men must rely on gender-specific versions of this distinction, and, as a result, egg and sperm donors can construct different definitions of their connection to offspring. Men cannot help but see themselves as fathers, because they are providing sperm in a culture that equates male genetics with parenthood. Women can define themselves as not-mothers, because they are providing eggs in a culture in which it is possible to separate female genetics from parenthood. This is more than just a possibility for egg donors, though; it is a necessity given the censure of "bad mothers."

People who donate eggs and sperm say that one of the questions they hear most often is "What does it feel like to have kids running around out there?" The fact is women and men will answer this question in different ways. It is not that egg donors feel no connection whatsoever. Like sperm donors, they are willing to meet with offspring in the future and are even curious to see who they become. But for women, the defining connection is with recipients, not offspring. The opposite is true of sperm donors, who feel little connection to recipients but experience a defining connection to offspring.

Conclusion

As the technologies of artificial insemination and *in vitro* fertilization rendered eggs and sperm transferable from donor to recipient, markets developed for these bodily goods. In the earliest sperm donation programs, physicians organized donation as a quick task to be performed in exchange for cash, yet those running the first egg donation programs constructed the exchange as a gift from caring donor to grateful recipient. For most of the twentieth century, physicians retained control over the process of selecting donors, but in the late 1980s, they began to cede this task to commercial agencies. In sperm donation, this was a result of logistical difficulties associated with the transition to frozen sperm in the wake of the AIDS epidemic. In egg donation, physicians could not keep up with the rising demand as IVF with donor eggs became increasingly popular. However, even as the market expanded, the gendered understandings of donation originally mobilized by these physicians continued to appear in new and different organizational contexts: donation programs located in different parts of the country and driven by different missions, including feminist nonprofits, university clinics, and commercial agencies.

Venturing inside these contemporary programs, talking with staff, and hearing from donors reveals the myriad ways in which framing donation as a gift or a job influences day-to-day practices. At every stage of the donation process, egg agencies emphasize the connection between donor and recipient. Eggs cannot yet be frozen (unlike sperm), so an egg donor will cycle with "her" recipient, which lends a sense of camaraderie even if they never meet. In contrast, sperm bank staffers rarely mention recipients, and men produce samples that are stored for six months before being shipped all over the world. Donation programs pay women more than men because of the different levels of risk associated with IVF and masturbation, but this confluence of biology and technology does not explain why women receive a negotiated sum regardless of bodily performance and men receive standardized payments doled out every two weeks.

Nor are the particulars of the exchange determined by biology or technology. Theoretically, sperm banks could sell all of a donor's samples to "his" recipient (and indeed some banks do offer such "exclusivity" for a price), and there is no technological barrier to splitting eggs from one donor among several recipients. Sperm banks could emphasize the deep significance of the gift that men are giving, sharing details about recipients' lives with sperm donors, and passing on thank-you notes. Egg agencies could treat women like employees, paying them based on the number of eggs they produce and refraining from mentioning any details about the program's customers. But this is not how it works in the market for sex cells, where a woman's donation is considered a precious gift and a man's donation a job well done.

More than just influencing program protocols, these gendered understandings affect women's and men's experiences of paid donation, because organizing it as a gift or a job simultaneously encourages and discourages particular conceptualizations of the monetary exchange. Most women are drawn by the prospect of making money, but as they interact with staff and sometimes with recipients, they begin to define donation in terms of being compensated to help people have children. Egg donors are paid to undergo the shots and surgery associated with IVF, and as they are not attempting a long-awaited pregnancy, they have a less intense bodily experience of this technology than would be expected. Moreover, they are paid for completing the *process* of donation, not on the basis of its outcome (number of eggs), so when they talk about "giving enough," it is about making sure the recipients have a good chance at becoming pregnant. At the same time, egg donors downplay the significance of their genetic contribution. When a woman calls her donation "just an egg," she is removing herself from any suspicion of being a bad mother, the kind who would sell her baby, and underscoring her contribution to the recipient's motherhood project, a contribution that she defines as a "huge gift."

Most sperm donors, too, are attracted by the idea of making money, but their interactions with staff are more closely aligned to those of employees in a workplace. Clocking in at the bank on a regular basis, men must produce high-count samples, and they hear little about recipients. As a result, sperm donors conceptualize donation as a job, and the fact that payment is based on bodily performance leaves them feeling like "assets" or "resources" for the sperm bank. Drawing on broader cultural understandings of paternity, they offer straightforward definitions of themselves as fathers to offspring, a view that is only reinforced by the banks' identity-release programs, which mark as significant the *donor's* contribution, not what he is doing for the recipient.

In this market, gendered cultural norms of maternal femininity and paternal masculinity operate in complicated ways, some of which seem almost contradictory. Relying on such norms, egg agencies recruit women who express altruistic motivations that are consistent with nurturing caregiving, but staffers expect donors to stop short of actually seeing themselves as mothers. Sperm banks frame donation as a job, reflecting cultural expectations that men be productive breadwinners, but they, too, do not want sperm donors defining themselves as fathers who will be responsible for offspring. These organizational practices result from the *selective* mobilization of gendered ideals, with egg agencies and sperm banks drawing on some elements of maternal femininity and paternal masculinity to manage donors. And it is the confluence of those organizational practices with the broader cultural norms that lead sperm donors to simultaneously see themselves as fathers and feel like "assets," while egg donors can simultaneously consider their donation to be "just an egg" and a "huge gift."

This sociological rendering of the market for eggs and sperm contrasts with the traditional vision of a market offered by commodification scholars, a vision in which the monetary exchange is all that matters. It is the "underlying activity," and all the other factors that go into making a market—who is doing the buying and selling, what is being bought and sold, how the exchange is organized, and how the participants experience it—are dismissed as irrelevant.[1] But these factors *do* matter. The market for sex cells reveals that the gendered framing of donation as a gift or a job is enormously powerful in shaping the social process of bodily commodification, both in terms of how it is organized and experienced.

WHY?

The question that remains is why sperm donation is considered a job and egg donation a gift. To answer this question, I return to some of the themes from the Introduction regarding the relationship between economy and society and how the social relations within and between them are suffused with gendered norms. Specifically, I contend that a powerful cultural distinction between the market and the family generates underlying mechanisms that drive much of the organization and experience of the market for sex cells.

Traditionally, markets have been associated with paid work, and the family has been associated with private life. The prevailing image has been one of "separate spheres," in which there is a bright line between the public sphere of the market and the private sphere of the home. According to the traditional division of labor, men dominated the public sphere, leaving the home each day to go to work, where they earned money to provide for the family. Women reigned over the private sphere, bearing and nurturing children while maintaining the home and family ties. Even as these gender norms became less hegemonic—more and more women are joining the workforce, and more and more men are performing household duties—the association of men with the market and women with the family has persisted.

More than these gendered associations, though, the idea that market and family *should* be separate has survived enormous social changes during the course of the last century. In different times and places, the line between these spheres has been drawn in different ways, and the actual lines are rarely as distinct as they appear in the abstract.[2] However, the dichotomies that undergird this cultural distinction—public/private, work/home, and male/female—remain incredibly powerful in structuring social practices.

In effect, the market for sex cells collapses the distinction between the public sphere of the market and the private sphere of the home, because it is *family* that is *for sale*. Certainly, the staff in donation programs would never put it so bluntly, and economists might identify the actual product as eggs or sperm or the donors who provide them. But what those cells and donors make possible is families. Consequently, there is a deep tension between what is for sale and what is culturally appropriate, tension that both egg agencies and sperm banks manage by deploying the altruistic rhetoric of donation.

Furthermore, given that women are more closely associated with the home and family life, paid egg donation is a more direct violation of the cultural distinction between market and family than is paid sperm donation. Historically, men's relationship to the home has been defined in terms of being a breadwinner, of providing financially for the family, so the connection between monetary exchange and family life that exists in sperm banks does not pose the same "threat" that it does in egg agencies. As Sharon Hays puts it, the relationship between mother and child is "understood as more distant and more protected from market relationships than any other."[3] As a result, it is not only the language of donation that appears in egg agencies, but also the language of the gift, which serves to manage the cultural tension of women being paid for eggs that become children and create families.

The historical data suggest that the language of donation and, for women, the language of the gift, were present from the inception of the market. From the first physician–researchers experimenting with IVF to egg agencies in different parts of the country, egg donation is a gift, a compensated gift, but a gift. The paid provision of sperm has consistently been referenced as donation, but sperm banks do not put much effort into defining this donation as altruistic. I do not wish to suggest that these are conscious strategies, that such language was adopted at some staff meeting somewhere and then became systematic policy. It was present from the beginning and has appeared throughout the history of the market because it *makes sense*, culturally speaking.

Until now, the working assumption has been that biological differences between women and men fully account for the differences in the market for eggs and sperm. In contrast, the explanation offered here takes into account biology but draws on the cultural meanings associated with sex differences to contend that gendered expectations of women and men, particularly those around reproduction and the family, also contribute to creating a market where sperm donors are paid piecework wages on the basis of bodily production and egg donors are compensated for giving a priceless gift.

BODILY COMMODIFICATION AS SOCIAL PROCESS

This book serves as an extended call to refine the concept of bodily commodification. In this section, I draw on insights from the medical market for sex cells to propose a sociological approach to thinking about what happens when people are paid for bodily goods and services.

First, it is crucial to view commodification of the body as an interactive social process, one that occurs over time between people who occupy particular social locations. This contrasts with the prevailing view of commodification in bioethical writings, which is essentially that of a light switch: if money is exchanged, then there is commodification, and the author does not need to know much more than that to speculate about its objectifying, alienating, and dehumanizing effects. I argue that identifying the monetary exchange is just the first step in a rigorous analysis.

Second, given that bodily commodification is a social process, scholars should expect to find variation in how that process unfolds. The potential causes and effects of this variation are numerous and are likely to be related to the good or service being exchanged. At a minimum, researchers should be attuned to:

- the broader social context, including the historical time in which the exchange occurs, the space in which it is managed, and the cultural norms that influence it;
- the social and biological characteristics of those participating as buyers, brokers, and sellers;
- the extent to which each participant has access to different forms of social power and social control;
- the supply of and demand for the good and any regulations that govern its exchange; and
- the characteristics of the good itself, including whether it is present in all kinds of bodies, if it is renewable, if it is separable from the rest of the body, and if its provision entails risk.

Third, it is important to attend to at least two levels of analysis when examining variation in bodily commodification: the organization of the market and the experiences of those participating in the market. Given the dominant assumption that commodification is commodification is commodification, scholars have paid little attention to variation in how markets for bodily goods and services are organized. Social scientists have begun some of the detailed, empirical work to trace this variation, but it is still rare to find comparative, qualitative data from buyers, brokers, and sellers about their experiences in different kinds of markets. As a result, the primary question asked in this book suggests a new angle on bodily commodification: how does variation in the organization of markets shape the experiences of participants in those markets?

Answering this question reveals one of the significant findings from this study: the way in which payment happens (i.e., *how* the money is handed over) is surprisingly important in shaping egg and sperm donors' experiences of being paid for bodily goods. Thus, the fourth and final suggestion for refining the concept of bodily commodification is to pay extremely close attention to the monetary exchange itself, both in terms of what the money is called and how it is doled out. Is the money referred to as a gift or compensation, as income or wages, or something else? Who refers to it that way? Do those who organize the market and those who participate in it call the money the same thing? When and how is the money paid? Is it all at once, or is it based on the provision of particular goods or the completion of particular acts? Each detail is not necessarily significant on its own, but together they reveal underlying assumptions about what kind of market it is and what kinds of social relationships are appropriate.

Each of the four elements in this proposal stresses the necessity of systematic, empirical research on markets for bodily goods rather than relying on abstract distinctions between gifts and commodities or between the family and the market. Learning more about how markets for bodily goods and services work in practice will offer a way out of interminable debates about whether commodification is objectifying or liberating, dehumanizing or empowering, because normative questions such as these cannot be answered *a priori*. Commodification is not a generic or uniform process, and it can result in different kinds of outcomes for different kinds of people in different kinds of situations.

In sum, debates about bodily commodification need to be infused with a more detailed understanding of what actually happens when people are paid for parts of their bodies. Much remains to be learned about the interactional dynamics in such markets, of how subtle and not so subtle differences in framing the exchange influence how each party responds to the transaction. Moreover, comparative research is also necessary to examine how the setting of such exchanges—in medical clinics, on the black market, and in countries with more and less regulation—matters. Social scientists working in this arena need to analyze precisely how it is that the structure and experience of bodily commodification is shaped by social categories and social inequalities, as economic valuations intertwine with cultural norms in specific organizational contexts.

BIOLOGICAL FACTORS IN SOCIOLOGICAL ANALYSES

This book also contributes to debates among social scientists about how to assess the role of biology in social processes. Feminists have historically avoided biological explanations, which is understandable given the regularity with which sex differences are referenced to deflect criticism of social inequalities. But decades of research on women's disadvantages do not lead one to expect a market in which women are more valued than men and where having a child can actually make a woman a more desirable candidate. These unexpected findings are explained, however, once the body is taken into account, both in its materiality, including differentiated reproductive organs, and in the meanings associated with this differentiated materiality, such as economic interpretations (e.g., eggs as a scarce resource) and cultural readings (e.g., women as nurturing).

Thus, as Judith Butler theorizes, the body does matter, but biology does not provide a set of static facts to be incorporated into sociological analyses, because biological factors alone do not predict any particular outcome. Indeed, empirical investigations into the meaning of reproductive cells and bodies reveal considerable variation in different social contexts. For example, Emily Martin finds that metaphors in medical textbooks privilege male bodies. However, in the medical market for eggs and sperm, some of these same "biological facts" result in higher monetary compensation and more cultural validation for women—validation that is based on a different set of gendered stereotypes about caring femininity and breadwinning masculinity.

But it is not only gender that influences the valuation of sex cells. Donation programs have difficulty recruiting diverse donors, so Asian and African American women might be paid a few thousand dollars more, and sperm banks reported relaxing height restrictions to accommodate Asian and Hispanic men. This paradoxical finding, that women of color are often compensated at higher levels for their reproductive material than are white women, is illuminated by intersectionality theory, which contends that gender, race, and class can combine in unpredictable ways, sometimes resulting in advantage or disadvantage depending on the social context.[4] In this market, race and ethnicity are biologized, as in references to Asian eggs or Jewish sperm, and these are some of the primary sorting mechanisms in donor catalogs, along with hair and eye color. This routinized reinscription of race at the genetic and cellular level in donation programs, which as medicalized organizations offer a veneer of scientific credibility to such claims, is worrisome given our eugenic history.[5]

In sum, it is essential for sociologists to attend to biological factors while simultaneously resisting essentialized biological explanations. Although reproductive cells and reproductive bodies are the salient biological factors in this market, sociologists working in other contexts are likely to encounter assumptions about other kinds of bodily difference. Incorporating biological factors into sociological analyses can also mean measuring the physical effects of gendered expectations. For example, although Arlie Hochschild discusses the biological basis of emotion, she does not focus on the biological *consequences* of different kinds of emotional labor. She concludes that female flight attendants experience more cognitive dissonance than do male debt collectors, but the long-term biological effects of manufactured smiling may actually be less severe than those of manufactured anger, which has clear cardiovascular implications.[6] In another example of physical effects, it is important for sociologists to explore how embodied experiences can vary by social context, as in egg donors' blasé descriptions of IVF and sperm donors' fluctuating sperm counts. There remains much work to be done in specifying the mechanisms through which the bodies of those who make markets interact with other cultural, economic, and structural factors in shaping those markets.

MARKETS FOR BODILY GOODS

In this section, I turn to markets for other kinds of bodily goods and briefly consider how the findings from this book might shed new light on the trade in blood, organs, surrogacy, and sex.[7] Specifically, I draw attention to the ways in which the market for eggs and sperm in the United States is both like and unlike markets for these other goods and services, including the extent to which each good is associated with the gender of the provider, whether providers receive direct payment, and whether the monetary exchange is stigmatized and/or legal.

Comparing how eggs and sperm are commodified highlights the importance of gendered cultural norms in structuring the organization and experience of the market for sex cells, but it is an open question whether such norms play such a significant role in markets for other bodily goods. For example, blood and organs are not sexed bodily goods in the same way that eggs and sperm are. They certainly come from male and female bodies and are transferred into male and female bodies, but blood and organs from a female can usually be transferred into a male and vice versa. However, this does not mean that gender norms are insignificant. To give just one example, scholars in Germany recently took up the long-identified gender discrepancy in living kidney donation in which women are more likely to be donors and men are more likely to be recipients. They found that part of the discrepancy is due to the fact that *mothers* donate to their children more often than do *fathers* and conclude by pointing to the power of gendered expectations, especially those of women as caregivers to children, in swaying decisions to donate.[8]

Another contrast is that, unlike egg and sperm donors, blood and organ donors in the United States are generally not paid, though there is a thriving secondary market among medical professionals for these goods. Kieran Healy's research clearly demonstrates the importance of organizational variation in shaping markets for blood and organs.[9] His findings raise an interesting question, however, about whether such variation results in different experiences for donors, particularly compared with countries that *do* allow direct payments or where black markets exist.[10] Consider the following two hypothetical kidney providers. The first is a poor man living in a shantytown in a developing country. He is paid $3,000 cash for one of his kidneys, which is removed in unsanitary conditions and transferred to a wealthy medical tourist. The second is a middle-class American man living in the suburbs. He is given a $3,000 credit toward health insurance for agreeing to donate his kidneys after his death. Both of these men and their kidneys are commodified, yet the organization and experience of the market is likely to be dramatically different. This seems obvious, but, in fact, bioethical treatments of commodification would generally lump these sorts of examples together because of the simple fact that monetary value has been assigned to part of the human body.

In both surrogate motherhood and prostitution, there is no question that gender norms are important in shaping market processes, but there is significant variation in how it is that gender matters. For example, recent ethnographic studies of surrogacy in Israel and India reveal differences in the commodification of gestation that depend in part on how gift rhetoric intertwines with ideals of motherhood and economic necessity in each national context.[11] My explanation for the dynamics at play in the American market for sex cells might not hold in other contexts. However, it does seem to hold for the surrogacy market in the United States, where the practice of paying women to carry a pregnancy continues to be controversial, so much so that some states have prohibited payments or banned the practice altogether. Even more than egg donors, surrogates risk being portrayed as mothers who hand over children for cash, and indeed, social scientists have documented the same "gift of life" rhetoric among surrogacy agencies, surrogate mothers, and their recipients.[12]

Although men cannot (yet) be surrogates, they can be prostitutes. However, as in egg and sperm donation, there are few studies that directly compare male and female sex work. When considered together, though, studies on particular aspects of the sex trade suggest it, too, exhibits significant variation in the organization and experience of the market, both by the gender of the provider and the gender of the consumer, as well as race, class, sexuality, and nationality. For example, Trevon Logan culled quantitative data from a national website advertising male escorts in the United States and found that the men serve a wide range of customers, from gay-identified men to heterosexually-identified men. Those who advertise more "masculine" behaviors charge higher prices for their services.[13] In a different national context, Don Kulick's ethnographic study of Brazilian *travestis* reveals how masculinity and sexuality come together to create a market in which people who are born with male genitalia dress as women and have sex with men for both money and pleasure.[14] Turning to female prostitution, Elizabeth Bernstein's comparative research in San Francisco, Amsterdam, and Sweden traces the shifting structure of this market over the past several decades. In particular, she considers how such changes have affected the embodied experiences of sex workers. Bernstein also finds inspiration in Viviana Zelizer's research, and she concludes with a call for closer empirical attention to variation in such markets. "Rather than taking commodification to be a self-evident totality, . . . I stress the ethical necessity of distinguishing *between* markets for sexual labor, based on the social location and defining features of any given type of exchange."[15]

Now, in contrast to markets for blood, organs, and surrogacy, altruistic rhetoric does not appear to be a salient feature of the market for sex. It is difficult to imagine male or female prostitutes claiming to be "donors" of sex, which raises the question of when it is that gift talk and bodily commodification can coexist. In keeping with the significance of gender, gift rhetoric may be more likely to appear, and to be more "sticky," when it comes to bodily goods that women donate because of cultural ideals of women as caring and selfless. Along the same lines, production rhetoric may appear more often for goods that men donate. However, this still does not explain why gift rhetoric does not appear in female prostitution. Lesley Sharp suggests that gift talk and bodily commodification are especially likely to coexist in medical settings, and that would certainly hold for the cases discussed here (blood, organs, and surrogacy versus prostitution).[16] Another potential explanation is that prostitution does not violate the market/family divide in quite the same way as egg donation and surrogacy, markets in which children are being created.

This book has focused on how gendered norms influence the market for sex cells, but as is clear from several of the examples in this section, racial and class-based inequalities, among others, are likely to be just as powerful in shaping processes of bodily commodification. Little is known about when and how various social categories come to matter in markets for bodily goods, but one area where there have been several detailed empirical studies is the use of racial categories in the field of genetics.[17] As Rayna Rapp points out, it is the newest technologies that seem to attract the oldest stereotypes.[18]

SEX CELLS

Sex does indeed sell in the medical market for eggs and sperm. Inside every reproductive cell are tightly coiled strands of DNA, and the value of this genetic material is understood through the lens of the donor's biological sex. Those who work to maintain this market, from buyers and brokers to sellers and regulators, calibrate their actions in ways that align with cultural norms of maternal femininity and paternal masculinity. The result is a classic evocation of the gendered division of labor: women's bodies are managed though the emotional work of caring about recipients, and men's bodies are regulated via a paycheck conditioned on sperm count. Nevertheless, this classic evocation produces surprising results. Women are paid much more than men, but the connection they establish with recipients, along with the availability of gift rhetoric, forestalls other potential understandings of remunerated donation, such as being paid for body parts. Men are not encouraged to feel any such connection with recipients, so although they are exempt from this form of emotional labor, the result is that they experience paid donation as a job, which leads to feelings of objectification and alienation. Whether eggs or sperm, blood or organs, surrogacy or sex, the social process of assigning economic value to the human body is the result of a confluence of factors. The characteristics of the people and the parts, the flows of supply and demand, and the historical and cultural context all come together to produce variation in both the structure and experience of the market.

APPENDIX A Egg and Sperm Donors'
Characteristics at Time
of Interview

Name	Program	Interview Year	Age	Egg: Cycles Sperm: Visits / Week	Education	Marital Status	Race/Ethnicity	Identity-Release	Met Recipients	No. of Own Children
					WOMEN					
Carla	CB	2002	25	1.5	Pursuing BA	Married	Hispanic, White		No	1
Jane	CB	2002	19	3	Pursuing BA	Single	Asian		Yes	0
Megan	CB	2002	22	1	Pursuing BA	Single	White		Yes	0
Olivia	CB	2002	23	4.5	Pursuing BA	Single	African American, White		Yes	0
Samantha	CB	2002	24	2	BA	Single	Hispanic, White		No	0
Tiffany	CB	2002	25	0	Some college	Divorced	White		Yes	0
Beth	OC	2002	31	6	Unknown	Single	White		Yes	0
Kim	OC	2002	23	0	BA	Single	White		No	0
Lisa	OC	2002	26	2	Some college	Separated	White		No	2
Nicole	OC	2002	35	4	BA	Single	African American, Hispanic, White		Yes	1
Rosa	OC	2002	32	2	Pursuing AA	Married	Hispanic		Yes	4
Gretchen	UFS	2006	26	2	BA	Single	White		Yes	0
Heather	UFS	2006	22	1	Pursuing BA	Single	White		No	0
Dana	GI	2006	25	4	AA	Married	White		No	3
Erica	GI	2006	27	2	Some college	Married	White		No	2
Jessica	GI	2006	30	1	BA	Married	White		No	0
Pam	GI	2006	27	2.5	Pursuing BA	Married	White		No	0
Susan	GI	2006	24	2	Some college	Divorced	White		No	1
Valerie	GI	2006	22	2	Pursuing AA	Single	White		No	0

Name		Year	Age		Education	Marital	Race			
Andrew	WS	2002	28	2	Pursuing PhD	Single	White	Yes	No	0
Ben	WS	2002	26	2	MA	Single	White	No→Yes	No	0
Dennis	WS	2002	24	2	BA	Single	White	Yes	No	0
Ethan	WS	2002	39	3	Pursuing MA	Married	White	Yes	No	0
Joe	WS	2002	46	Unk.	BA	Married	White	Yes	No	0
Manuel	WS	2002	27	3	Pursuing BA	Engaged	Asian, Hispanic	Yes	No	0
Brian	GI	2006	33	2	Unknown	Single	White	No	No	0
Charles	GI	2006	29	Var.	Pursuing MA	Single	White	Yes	No	0
Fred	GI	2006	22	2	Pursuing BS	Single	White	No	No	0
Greg	GI	2006	21	2	Pursuing BA	Single	White	Yes	No	0
Isaac	GI	2006	22	3	Pursuing BA	Engaged	Asian, Hispanic	Yes	No	0
Kyle	GI	2006	22	3	Pursuing AA	Single	White	Yes	No	0
Mike	GI	2006	22	3	Pursuing AA	Single	White	Yes	No	0
Nathan	GI	2006	38	2	Some college	Single	Hispanic, White	Yes	Yes	0
Paul	GI	2006	20	1	Pursuing BA	Single	White	Yes	No	0
Ryan	GI	2006	40	1	MA	Married	White	Yes	No	1
Scott	GI	2006	32	2	BA	Married	White	Yes	No	3
Travis	GI	2006	30	2	BS, MBA	Single	White	Yes	No	0
Victor	GI	2006	23	3	AA	Single	White	Yes	No	0
Walt	GI	2006	19	2	AA	Single	White	Yes	No	0

Demographics of Donors Based on Profiles at Egg and Sperm Donation Programs

	Women				Men			
	OVACORP	GAMETES INC.	CREATIVE BEGINNINGS	UNIVERSITY FERTILITY SERVICES	CRYOCORP	GAMETES INC.	WESTERN SPERM BANK	UNIVERSITY FERTILITY SERVICES
Number of Profiles	466	75	129	149	125	112	44	57
Year Profiles Collected	2002	2006	2002	2006	2002	2006	2002–2003	2006
Race/Ethnicity								
White	83%	73%	73%	91%	74%	79%	68%	95%
Asian	2%	0%	12%	0%	17%	5%	9%	2%
Hispanic	7%	5%	7%	7%	3%	4%	7%	4%
African American	8%	21%	5%	3%	5%	10%	7%	0%
Multiple	0%	0%	4%	0%	2%	1%	9%	0%
Age at Profile								
Mean	28	25	22	26	24	26	27	25
Min, Max.	20, 34	20, 33	18, 31	21, 34	19, 38	18, 38	19, 40	19, 38
Standard Deviation	3.6	3.6	2.9	3.4	4.1	5.1	6.6	4.8
Ages 18–22	9%	35%	53%	22%	38%	34%	39%	33%
Ages 23–27	40%	40%	34%	47%	40%	31%	23%	42%
Ages 28–40	50%	25%	5%	31%	22%	33%	39%	25%
Missing	1%	0%	7%	0%	0%	2%	0%	0%
Education								
High School Only	6%	4%	12%	11%	0%	4%	2%	0%†
Some College	48%	67%	64%	62%	45%	45%	50%	35%
Bachelor's Degree	19%	27%	24%	21%	41%	43%	39%	46%
Graduate Degree	6%	3%	1%	4%	14%	8%	9%	7%
Missing	20%	0%	0%	1%	0%	0%	0%	12%

Occupation								
Student	11%	67%	53%	52%	58%	40%	57%	72%
Nonstudent	80%	31%	40%	38%	42%	59%	43%	7%
Homemaker	8%	3%	5%	8%	0%	0%	0%	0%
Missing	1%	0%	2%	1%	0%	1%	0%	21%
Marital Status								
Single	38%	N/A	80%	56%	N/A	71%	N/A	77%
Married	48%	N/A	17%	36%	N/A	25%	N/A	19%
Divorced	14%	N/A	2%	8%	N/A	4%	N/A	2%
Missing	0%	N/A	1%	0%	N/A	0%	N/A	2%
Has Own Children	71%	36%	21%	38%	N/A	21%	N/A	18%
Identity-Release	N/A	N/A	N/A	N/A	N/A	36%	52%	N/A
Jewish	2%	0%	N/A	2%	2%	7%	16%	19%
Year Profile Completed								
Mean	2001	N/A	2001	1998	1999	2001	2001	1992
Min., Max.	1998–2002	N/A	2001–2002	1993–2006	1990–2002	1995–2005	1996–2003	1986–2001
Standard Deviation	0.9 yrs	N/A	0.5 yrs	3.2 yrs	3.6 yrs	2.3 yrs	1.7 yrs	4.4 yrs

Some columns might not total 100% because of rounding error. Data are culled from donor profiles. I visited the OvaCorp, Creative Beginnings, and CryoCorp websites once each in 2002 to gather data on all posted profiles. Because of the small number of profiles at Western Sperm Bank, I visited the program's website once in 2002 and a second time in 2003, gathering an additional 14 profiles. I visited the Gametes Inc. websites (there are separate sites for egg and sperm donors) once in 2006. University Fertility Services has very small donor programs. It does not post profiles online, so I looked through its paper files to gather donors' demographic information. Statistics for University Fertility Services include all men accepted to be sperm donors from 1986 to 2001 and all women accepted to be egg donors from 1993 to 2006.

† Educational level for University Fertility Services' sperm donors was sometimes difficult to determine because staffers updated the form based on the level of education the man eventually completed (e.g., a nineteen-year-old donor is listed as having a medical degree). I attempted to make these statistics conform with the other donation programs to the extent possible.

Notes

1. Debora Spar of the Harvard Business School (2006, 3) estimated revenues for each of the following components of the fertility industry in 2004: fertility drugs at $1,331,860,000; IVF at $1,038,528,000; diagnostic tests at $374,900,000; donor sperm at $74,380,000; donor eggs at $37,773,000; and surrogate mothers at $27,400,000 for a total of $2,884,841,000.

2. National statistics for sperm donation have not been generated since 1987, when the United States Office of Technology Assessment (1988) estimated that 30,000 children born that year had been conceived with donated sperm. For a discussion of the number of egg donation cycles per year, see Chapter 1.

3. One recent study reported an average payment of $4,200 per egg donation (Covington and Gibbons 2007).

4. On prostitution, see Bernstein (2007). On the medical profession's use of bodies and body parts to study anatomy, see Richardson (1987). Selling blood is not illegal, but most whole blood donors in the United States are not paid. Individuals do sell a part of blood called plasma (Espeland 1984), and sometimes

people with rare blood types are paid to provide blood. The National Organ Transplant Act makes it illegal to sell one's organs in the United States. However, for both blood and organs, there is a highly developed secondary market through which such goods are exchanged among medical professionals (Healy 2006, Timmermans 2006). On face transplants, see Talley (2008).

5. Over time, the inability to become pregnant has become defined as a "medical problem" through a process called medicalization, in which the medical profession gains authority to define conditions as requiring medical intervention (Conrad 2007). On the history of infertility, see Pfeffer (1993) and Becker (2000).

6. Women and men are equally likely to experience infertility, but incidence rates are based on women's responses to the National Survey of Family Growth. See Stephen and Chandra (2006), which reports an infertility rate of 7.4% among married women in 2002 and includes a discussion of social trends, including delayed marriage, delayed childbearing, and increasing educational attainment.

7. Mamo (2007).

8. On the history of insemination, see Sherman (1964), Daniels (2006), and Moore (2007). Sperm that is placed directly into a woman's uterus must be "washed" of all seminal fluid to prevent the uterus from expelling it. Sperm donation programs do this at the time of the donation, and they sell "washed" samples for slightly higher prices than regular samples.

9. In the 1930s, researchers John Rock and Miriam Menkin began to purposely schedule ovary removal surgeries when the patient would be ovulating. For six years, Menkin took each ovary back to the lab and looked for ripe eggs to mix with sperm. In 1944, they reported the first successful fertilization of sperm and egg in the lab (Duka and DeCherney 1994, 83). On the history of IVF, see Duka and DeCherney (1994) and Thompson (2005).

10. An increasing awareness of the problems associated with gestating multiple fetuses have led to calls for physicians to reduce the number of embryos transferred to the uterus (American College of Obstetrics and Gynecology 2006). Yet, American physicians retain wide latitude in how they practice, as is evident in the case of Nadya Suleman. In 2008, her physician transferred far more embryos than was standard practice, and she gave birth to eight children, which led to a media firestorm during which she was dubbed "Octomom" in headline after headline.

11. On surrogacy, see Ragoné (1994), Markens (2007), and Teman (2010). When surrogacy was first offered through commercial agencies in the early 1980s, the surrogate mother (the woman gestating the fetus) also provided the egg. This was the situation in the controversial "Baby M" case in 1987, in which Mary Beth

Whitehead provided the egg and gestational services for William and Mary Stern before reneging on the contract and seeking custody of the child. With the development of egg donation, it is now the case that most surrogate mothers are not genetically related to the fetuses they gestate (Ragoné 1998).

12.   Practice Committee of ASRM (2008b). Empirical studies have been conducted by Sauer (2001) and Maxwell, Cholst, and Rosenwaks (2008). According to ASRM, ovarian hyperstimulation occurs when "the ovaries become swollen and painful. Fluid may accumulate in the abdominal cavity and chest, and the patient may feel bloated, nauseated, and experience vomiting or lack of appetite." ASRM estimates that about a third of all women who take fertility medications will experience mild hyperstimulation, which is treated with over-the-counter painkillers and a reduction in activity. It estimates that around 1% will experience severe hyperstimulation, which can require hospitalization.

13.   Schneider (2008) and Elton (2009).

14.   See Haimes (1993) for a discussion of how gendered understandings of gamete donation shaped the initial regulatory deliberations in Britain.

15.   In 1984, ASRM created an ethics committee to investigate the ramifications of IVF. Committee members included physicians, lawyers, ethicists, biologists, and a priest. The first ethics report was issued in 1986, and follow-up reports have been generated every few years (Duka and Decherney 1994, 188).

16.   See, for example, Landes and Posner (1978) on adoption markets and Becker and Elias (2007) on organ markets.

17.   Titmuss (1971, 158).

18.   Murray (1996, 62).

19.   Nussbaum (1998, 695).

20.   Titmuss (1971, 245–6).

21.   Zelizer (1979), Zelizer (1985), and Zelizer (2005).

22.   Zelizer (1988, 618). As Zelizer's theoretical project is most developed in the commodification of intimate relationships, such as those between husband and wife or parent and child, this analysis of the medical market for sex cells builds on her work by examining the intimate processes of bodily commodification among those who did not previously know each other. My research also differs from Zelizer's in its focus on particular bodily goods as opposed to the commodification of whole persons.

23.   Radin (1996, xiii).

24.   Healy (2006, 120). Emphasis in original. Healy's research is part of a trend in economic sociology toward empirical studies of markets (e.g., Baker [1984], Abolafia [1996], and Velthuis [2005]), but it is one of the few empirical studies of markets for bodily goods.

25.   See De Beauvoir (1989), Ortner (1974), and Rubin (1975).

26. Yanagisako and Collier (1990, 132).

27. Butler (1993). See also Fausto-Sterling (2000).

28. Martin (1991, 500).

29. For a review, see England and Folbre (2005).

30. Nelson and England (2002, 1). On public/private as a fractal distinction, see Gal and Kligman (2000). On gendered norms of parenthood, see Chodorow (1978), Connell (1987), Hays (1996), Coltrane (1996), Blair-Loy (2003), and Kimmel (2006).

31. Appadurai (1986, 11–12). See Marx (1936) and Mauss (1967). On the distinction between commodities and gifts, see Rubin (1975), Gregory (1982), and Carrier (1995).

32. Sharp (2000, 292).

33. Radin differentiates "market rhetoric" from actual buying and selling and discusses the power of such rhetoric (1996, 104).

34. Scheper-Hughes (2001b, 2). Emphasis added.

35. Hochschild (1983). See, for example, Kanter (1977), Acker (1990), Pierce (1995), Williams (1995), Hondagneu-Sotelo (2001), Sherman (2007), and Otis (2008).

36. Lopez (2006, 137).

37. The bioethical literature often provides examples of individual experiences, commonly drawn from newspaper reports, but this does not constitute systematic research on the experience of commodification. Radin (1996) points to the possibility of variation in how payment is experienced, but she did not collect empirical data. Waldby and Mitchell (2006) did not collect data from donors. Titmuss (1971) and Healy (2006) did analyze data from blood and/or organ donors but in the form of surveys and not qualitative interviews and observation. Bernstein (2007) includes an analysis of the embodied experience of commodification, but it is a study of sex workers.

38. See, for example, Jordan (1983), Gordon (1976), Luker (1984), Katz Rothman (1986), Ragoné (1994), Ginsburg and Rapp (1995), Browner and Press (1995), Franklin (1997), Roberts (1997), Kligman (1998), Beisel and Kay (2004), Markens (2007), and Teman (2010).

39. Sharp (2000).

40. This sample of six donation programs is limited in three ways. First, it is not a random sample of all donation programs in the United States, a selection strategy that, although ideal, would be difficult to enact because there is no comprehensive list of all such programs. Second, this sample does not capture data about "private" donation, which takes place within family and friendship networks or through contacts made on the Internet. Systematic recruitment of these subjects would be difficult, but more importantly for the theoretical project of analyzing variation in commodification, donors to family and friends are rarely paid,

and the influence of personal relationships would be difficult to analyze separately from the experience of providing genetic material. In terms of Internet donation, few men participate, which makes a gendered comparison difficult. Thus, I limited my project to analyzing variation in bodily commodification within the formalized structure of organized donation programs. Third, in focusing on the staff and donors at organized donation programs, I did not collect data about recipients, who, as consumers of reproductive technologies, create demand for eggs and sperm. Instead, I draw on existing research about how recipients make decisions about donors and how those decisions are influenced by staff at organized donation programs (e.g. Becker 2000; Becker, Butler, and Nachtigall 2005).

41.   In most cases, I simply cold-called the program, identifying myself as a graduate student interested in learning about egg and sperm donation. The exceptions include Creative Beginnings, which is run by the mother of a fellow graduate student, and University Fertility Services, where my parents' neighbor used to run the egg donation program. After interviewing the first person I contacted in each program, I requested to speak with other staff, and eventually I asked to interview donors.

At OvaCorp in 2002, I interviewed the donor manager, several of her assistants, and two psychologists who screen donors. I spent one day observing at the program's offices, which included attending a weekly staff meeting with the agency director, a psychologist, a lawyer, the donor manager, and an assistant. I re-interviewed one of the OvaCorp psychologists in 2006, because she was instrumental in starting its egg donation program after working for several years on the surrogacy side. At Creative Beginnings in 2002, I interviewed every member of the staff, including the founder/executive director, assistant director, financial manager, office manager, and several office assistants. I also observed for six days in the program's offices and attended two of their informational meetings for women interested in egg donation.

In sharp contrast to the egg agencies, it was more difficult to gain access to the sperm banks. (Schmidt and Moore [1998] also point to this kind of "organizational gatekeeping," which is probably related to the emphasis on anonymity in sperm donation, which I discuss in Chapter 1). In 2002, I interviewed Cryo-Corp's marketing director, who also gave me a tour of the bank, but I was denied access to other staff. After a 2005 interview with a prominent physician–researcher who said I could use his name, I contacted the founder/medical director of CryoCorp. At the conclusion of my interview with him, I requested interviews with other members of his staff. He introduced me to the CEO, who granted final permission. In 2006, I interviewed the CEO, two recipient managers, two donor managers, a donor recruiter, a genetic counselor, and the human resources manager.

I encountered similar hesitancy at Western Sperm Bank when I first made contact in 2002. The staff asked for a detailed research plan, my résumé, and a writing sample. Interestingly, it was my work at a pro-choice organization before entering graduate school that eased their minds about my intentions as a researcher, and I was allowed to interview the donor manager, the research director, and a donor/recipient staff person. In 2004, I returned for a brief visit to interview the executive director and tour the sperm bank.

On my first research trip to University Fertility Services in 2005, I interviewed one of the physicians, the nurse responsible for egg donation, and the nurse responsible for sperm donation (among their many other duties). After completing Health Insurance Portability and Accountability Act (HIPAA) training and IRB review at that university (in addition to IRB review at my home institution), I returned for a longer trip in 2006 and talked again with the same physician and both nurses. I also interviewed the medical director, the psychologist, the embryologist, one of the lab technicians, and a third physician who worked in the practice but was part-time.

My two trips to Gametes Inc. in 2006 were organized in a similar way, with the first trip involving a three-hour interview with the founder/executive director and brief conversations with the egg and sperm donor managers. On the second, longer visit, I re-interviewed the donor managers and also spoke to the directors of clinical operations, finance, marketing, and shipping as well as several assistants and lab technicians. Gametes Inc. has two locations; "headquarters" is in a small city, and the satellite office is in a larger city a few hours away. I interviewed staff and observed at both locations.

Although it was sometimes difficult to get in, once I was granted access, staff members at all of the programs were unbelievably helpful and patient in responding to my many, many questions.

42.   I interviewed six sperm donors from Western Sperm Bank and fourteen sperm donors from Gametes Inc., half of whom donated at "headquarters" and half at the satellite office (see previous note). After extensive negotiations, Cryo-Corp agreed to put a sign-up sheet for interviews near the entrance the donors used, but after a week, there were no names on it. One staff member said she even personally asked her most gregarious donor, and he declined. She speculated that my affiliation with a university where many of the donors attended school might have contributed to their lack of interest. At University Fertility Services, the staff had not actively recruited sperm donors for several years, and they were not willing to contact past donors on my behalf. They thought the men would not be cooperative (previous attempts to contact former sperm donors about updating disease testing had not always been successful) and did not want to invade their privacy.

43. Previous studies suggest that sperm donors who release identifying information about themselves differ from those who wish to remain anonymous, both in terms of their initial motivations for donation as well as in their attitudes about offspring (Foster-Fraser 1990 and Daniels and Haimes 1998). So it is important for the reader to note that the findings reported here may reflect this selected population. It is also possible that their willingness to be known to offspring makes them more willing to be known to a researcher.

44. In general, the interviews I did in 2002 were much longer, averaging a little more than two hours for egg and sperm donors alike. By the time I began interviewing donors again in 2006, the interviews had become considerably more focused. This, combined with the fact that Gametes Inc. required me to interview donors in the program's offices, often when they had just dropped by to donate or take care of other paperwork, made the interviews shorter. Most of the remaining interviews were in restaurants or coffee shops. Three of the interviews with egg donors took place in the women's homes.

45. Codes for the donor interviews included:

- *Donor's Response to*: Ads/Recruitment; First Contact with Program; Screening/Profiles; Legal Contract; Confidentiality/Anonymity/Identity Release; Matching with Recipients; Abstinence; Bank Visits/Masturbation; Hormones/ Shots/Egg Retrieval; Being a Number; Repeated/Continued Donation; Gifts; Other.
- *Donor's Relationship to*: Staff; Money; Gametes/Offspring/Recipients; Own Reproductive History/Future; Other Donors; Other.
- *Donation as Compared to*: Job; Donating Other Body Parts; Surrogacy; Parenthood; Adoption; Other.
- *Donor's Rhetoric*: Helping/Gift/Service; Genetics; Science/Technology; Prochoice; Religious/Spiritual; Emotions; Programs as Businesses; Other.
- *Miscellaneous*: Donation as Part of Identity; Changing Views; Recommended Program Changes; Resistance to Program Policies; Summing up Experience; Other Programs; Telling Others about Donation.

I did not limit the number of codes that could be applied to a particular interview excerpt. In the end, each code contained anywhere from a few pages to 150 pages of interview excerpts, with the exception of Gametes/Offspring/Recipients, which was more than 300 pages long. I printed out each code as needed and did more detailed coding on paper. At the same time, I was also creating a spreadsheet that grew to include more than 300 variables about each donor's interview, including everything from their ages to whether they used specific words or phrases in discussing donation.

1. CHARACTERIZING THE MATERIAL

1. See Hard (1909), mentioned in Daniels (2006). In the article, Dr. Hard reports meeting the young man and shaking his hand, which has fueled speculation that he was in fact the donor.

2. Daniels (2006, 76).

3. Tompkins (1950).

4. Guttmacher et al. (1950, 266–268).

5. This is a reference to the eugenic logic of a previous generation that still held sway over the field (Daniels 2006).

6. Davis (1956).

7. Duka and DeCherney (1994, 65).

8. On medicalization, see Conrad (2007). On the history of the medical profession, see Freidson (1970) and Starr (1982). On the power of the medical profession in matters of reproduction, see Luker (1984) and Roberts (1997).

9. Several of the physicians I interviewed for this study were in their forties and fifties and remember being asked to donate sperm in medical school.

10. A 1938 article in *Time* magazine profiled the Georgetown University School of Medicine, where medical students and residents were paid $25 per sample (Daniels 2006, 79). By the mid-1980s, Novaes (1985, 576) notes that most sperm donors were still being paid between $20 and $35.

11. Guttmacher et al. (1950, 268).

12. See, for example, Murphy (1964), which details a study of 511 men who had applied to donate sperm at the Farris Institute for Parenthood in Philadelphia in the previous two decades. All of the applicants were students, with most enrolled in medical school. About a fifth were rejected for low sperm count and about half for other reasons with the remainder going on to donate, but the majority provided fewer than ten samples.

13. Titmuss (1971).

14. Guttmacher (1958, 370).

15. See Ansbacher (1978, 378). Scientists working on animal breeding in the 1860s were the first to propose "banks" to store frozen sperm, a project that eventually took hold, particularly in cattle breeding. Cryopreservation experiments with human sperm began in the 1930s, but it proved more fragile than bull sperm. It took several decades to render the technology successful in humans (Sherman 1964). The first children conceived with frozen and thawed sperm were born in 1953. Shortly thereafter, the first banks dedicated to storing human sperm opened in the United States, including the Tyler Clinic in Los Angeles. These banks were initially intended for men who wanted to freeze their own sperm as "insurance" against some future calamity or illness (Dan-

iels 2006, 81–90). Reproductive medicine, including artificial insemination and IVF, has a long history of exchanging ideas and techniques with veterinary medicine (Clarke 1998 and Friese 2009).

16.   Novaes (1985).

17.   Peterson (1986, 569).

18.   United States Office of Technology Assessment (1988, 10).

19.   Daniels (2006, 91).

20.   Daniels (2006, 90–91).

21.   However, if a physician requests that the sperm be shipped directly to a patient's home, then the sperm banks will do so.

22.   In a 2006 interview, the embryologist at University Fertility Services described current practices for assessing sperm.

> You normally expect at least a 50% recovery of sperm [after it is frozen and thawed], and therefore what you're looking for in a sperm donor is somebody that has high sperm counts, good motility, vigorous moving sperm, and you would like to have a known fertility status on the donor. You don't always know that. Certainly with the younger donors, that's not always assured. There used to be some testing that went along with the screening to at least try to get some indication of the fertility factor of the sperm, usually just based on sperm numbers and sperm count. Now we're adding sperm morphology, because morphology and function are very tightly connected with sperm. Everything is put together for one purpose, and that's transporting chromosomes, DNA. The sperm head is very dense and compact. It has some structure to it that you can see under certain conditions, which have to do with its ability to bind and transfer through that outer membrane of the egg zona. So that's something that can be assessed as well. Of course, the mid piece [of the sperm] is primarily concerned with the generation of the energy production, ATP [adenosine triphosphate], which drives the tail to drive the motility. So we can take account of all those things to give a morphological index, which then we presume will carry through to some kind of a functional ability. That's what we look for in a donor, and so they're highly selected.

23.   United States Office of Technology Assessment (1988, 9). Several interviewees at University Fertility Services mentioned a vote that the physicians and nurses in the practice had taken on this issue. The majority voted not to provide fertility services unless they were "medically necessary," which excluded single women and lesbians on the grounds that they did not have a medical diagnosis of infertility. In 2008, the California Supreme Court ruled that fertility practices could not discriminate on the basis of sexual orientation in *Benitez v. North Coast Women's Care Medical Group*.

24.   Scheib and Cushing (2007).

25.   Rosenwaks (1987). This article contains images of the technique being used in a cow and in a woman on opposing pages.

26.   Lutgen et al. (1984). As it became possible to freeze embryos in the late 1980s, the number of IVF patients willing to donate some of their eggs dwindled

(Kennard et al. 1989). One of the physician–researchers I interviewed in 2006 explained that this is

> still done in some centers, to have part of [a patient's IVF] expenses covered in exchange for donating some of the eggs. Most [centers] don't do that, partly because if she doesn't get pregnant, then that's difficult wondering if someone else got pregnant, and [she] was never able to have a child. The positive is that it can reduce the expenses for that patient. Most programs, because donors are so readily available, do egg donation with the donor.

There was also a third technique in use during the 1980s, one in which fertility programs relied on women undergoing tubal ligations to agree to take fertility medications. They would produce multiple eggs that could be retrieved at the same time as the sterilization surgery (Rosenwaks 1987).

27. Sauer et al. (1989).

28. Barad and Cohen (1996, 18).

29. Lessor et al. (1993, 66).

30. In one survey of fifty-two clinics providing egg donation in the early 1990s, nearly 80% required women to undergo psychological screening (Braverman 1993). Many of the physicians I interviewed were surprised to learn that sperm donors were not (and are not) psychologically screened.

31. Kennard et al. (1989, 660).

32. Nichols and Moore (2009). The article was picked up by several news outlets, including MSNBC and *Forbes* magazine.

33. Sauer and Paulson (1994).

34. Sauer and Paulson (1992). The survey included fifty-one clinics that offered egg donation in the early 1990s. Just about one-fifth of the clinics maintained a registry of donors, which listed between five and thirty-five women.

35. Braverman and Corson (1995, 543).

36. In the late 2000s, some programs and commercial firms began to offer egg-freezing services, but most of the physicians I interviewed in 2006 said that they did not believe that egg freezing was successful enough to warrant its use in clinical settings. See also Practice Committee of the ASRM (2008a).

37. This same physician described how his program had a leg up on the scientific competition, because they had managed to recruit a cohort of donors before others did. Here, the women willing to donate eggs and women willing to be recipients are catalogued alongside technology as necessary to medical innovation.

> There were, at that time, ten or so [academic] programs around the country that were interested in being at the forefront of the field and who moved along at approximately the same pace. We had a big advantage in that we had those donors, so we hit the ground running, and as soon as transvaginal egg retrieval became a reality, boom, we were ready to go. And we'd had patients that had already been recruited for that specifically, who had been lined up waiting to have it done. Most other

programs were not quite like that. They had to go through, "How are we going to recruit donors? Are we going to get this through the IRB? Is the research committee going to be interested in this?" All of those things take time.

38.   In the early 1990s, Sauer and Paulson (1992) contacted sixty-three clinics where ASRM referred patients interested in egg donation. Of the fifty-one respondents, one-fifth had not performed a single cycle, and two-thirds had performed fewer than ten cycles in the previous two years. Ten percent of the programs had performed more than one hundred cycles.

39.   Data come from the CDC's report *Assisted Reproductive Technology Success Rates* (2008). The CDC's statistics, which are based on an annual survey of fertility clinics, do not include information about who the donors are, so this latter figure probably includes donations from other IVF patients, relatives, friends, and paid donors. A more restrictive figure is the number of transfers involving fresh donor eggs (not all cycles end in a transfer of the embryo to the recipient), which hovers around 6–7% of all IVF cycles during this ten-year period, beginning at 3,822 transfers in 1996 and rising to 10,049 by 2006.

40.   Sauer and Paulson's (1992) study of fifty-one clinics reported donor fees ranging from $500 to $2,000. Around the same time, Braverman (1993) surveyed all SART members and found fifty-two programs that offered egg donation and paid donors between $750 and $3,500. Four programs used unpaid volunteers.

41.   Kennard et al. (1989) and Schover, Rothman, and Collins (1992).

42.   There do not appear to be any statistics available on the number of egg agencies over time. As of 2008, the ASRM listed ninety agencies in the United States that had agreed to abide by their guidelines governing egg donor compensation.

43.   Seibel and Kiessling (1993), Eastlund and Stroncek (1993), Sauer (1999) and Bergh (1999).

44.   Kolata (1998). In keeping with concerns about rising fees for egg donors, German et al. (2001) compared applicants to donation programs before and after the increase from $2,500 to $5,000. They found that women in the second group were more likely to finish their questionnaires, but there were not any significant differences in their social or epidemiological characteristics.

45.   Ethics Committee of the American Society for Reproductive Medicine (2000).

46.   Covington and Gibbons (2007). The list of approved egg agencies at *www.sart.org* is prefaced by the following statement: "These Egg Donor Agencies have all signed an agreement with the Society for Assisted Reproductive Technology (SART) that states that they will abide by the American Society for Reproductive Medicine (ASRM) Ethics Committee Guidelines governing the payment of egg donors. This information is self-reported and has not been verified by either ASRM or SART."

47. Hopkins (2006) and Rabin (2007). These debates have also spread into the realm of egg donation for stem cell research (Thompson 2007).

48. In total, fifty-seven men had been accepted as donors at University Fertility Services between 1986 and 2001.

49. The psychologist at OvaCorp described a similar situation at another university donation program. "We have a couple who wants to save money, so they're going to have the [university] IVF clinic find them a donor. Great, save a ton of money. It took four months to get a choice of one. Generic, nice, Caucasian girl, and they're fine with it, because that's who they are. It's cheaper, it's almost always anonymous, and it's totally doctor-controlled."

50. One extraordinary example of a university program gone awry comes from the University of California at Irvine. In 1995, the *Orange County Register* received the Pulitzer Prize for reporting on physicians there who were "donating" their patients' excess eggs without permission. There have also been scattered reports, as well as a few prosecutions, of fertility doctors surreptitiously using their own sperm to inseminate patients.

51. On the professional authority of physicians, see Freidson (1970) and Starr (1982). On the health care sector of the U.S. economy, see McKinley and Stoekle (1988) and Light (1993). On the women's health movement, see Bell (2009) and *Our Bodies, Ourselves,* first published in 1971, by the Boston Women's Health Book Collective. Physicians themselves also began to modify the definition of their role, shifting from the image provided in Guttmacher's 1955 statement, in which the doctor is responsible for evaluating both donor and recipient, to one in which the patients' reproductive choices are paramount. Thompson (2005) traces this historical process in the realm of IVF.

52. Relman (1980, 963).

2. SELLING GENES, SELLING GENDER

1. On the ways in which medicine is influenced by market forces, see Conrad and Leiter (2004), Light (2004), and McKinley and Stoekle (1988). On the cultural power of medical authority, see Parsons (1951), Freidson (1970), and Starr (1982).

2. Becker (2000) and Becker, Butler, and Nachtigall (2005). These studies are limited to heterosexual couples and do not include systematic comparisons of how recipients select egg donors versus sperm donors.

3. Rindfuss, Morgan, and Offutt (1996).

4. There is less screening of recipients. Creative Beginnings asks for recipients' health histories and doctors' names to confirm that they actually do "need" egg donation. OvaCorp and both sperm banks require certification that recipients are working with a doctor.

5. Being a "carrier" means that an individual has one copy of a defective gene that causes a disease but that person will not develop the disease. To develop the disease, a person must have two copies of the defective gene, one copy inherited from each biological parent. If both parents are carriers, there is a 25% chance the child will have cystic fibrosis and a 50% chance the child will be a carrier.

6. A study of attrition at Oregon Health Sciences University (OHSU) reports a similar rate (Gorrill et al. 2001). Researchers tracked all inquiries from potential egg donors for ten months in 1999. Of these, 315 women responded to the program's advertisements; 124 returned profiles; 82 were invited to an orientation session (the others were rejected based on age, weight, smoking, and/or family health history); 64 attended the orientation; and 56 began screening. Of those screened, 13 were rejected for medical or psychological reasons; 5 completed the screening but were lost despite follow-up efforts; and 38, or 12% of the women who initially inquired, entered the donor pool. OHSU estimated the cost of bringing one donor into the pool at $1,869.

7. Throughout its long history, donor insemination has been marked by extensive secrecy (see Chapter 1). CryoCorp and Western Sperm Bank do not share adult photos of sperm donors with recipients, but there are a few banks that do, including Gametes Inc.

8. The founder of another major egg agency on the West Coast had a similar response to online profiles. "The biggest change came with the Internet, because that made donors immediately available. It became a catalog for choosing people. It had the bonus that a lady from Australia can get online and see donors immediately [but] the detracting element of depersonalizing it and making the donors seem like a commodity or an object, rather than a person. So that was really hard."

9. It is not uncommon for egg agency staffers to refer to the donors as "girls."

10. See Almeling (2006) for an extended analysis of the donor profiles. To code altruistic and financial motivations, I categorized each donor's answer to the profile question "Why do you want to be a donor?" as reflecting an interest in "helping" and/or "money." In most cases, "helping" referred to the donor's interest in assisting recipients in having a child, but I also included donor responses as vague as "I get a good feeling knowing that I am helping others in some way." Most of the responses coded for "money" included explicit references to financial compensation, but I also included more vague references to donation as "mutually beneficial" for the donor and the recipient. Each donor's response was coded separately for "helping" and for "money."

11. Many of the physicians I interviewed for this study were surprised by the lengthy time commitment required of sperm donors, probably because the older sperm donation programs that were operating at the time they were in

medical school were not run in the same way (see Chapter 1). For example, in one mid-century study, the Farris Institute for Parenthood in Philadelphia reported that 60% of the men in the program had donated less than ten times. Just about a tenth had donated more than forty times (Murphy 1964).

12.   Ethics Committee of the American Society for Reproductive Medicine (2000).

13.   At some egg agencies, women are paid in two installments, the first (usually $1,000) when the donor begins injecting fertility medications and the remainder after the egg retrieval. Egg agencies do this so that the donor will receive some money even if the cycle is cancelled, usually as a result of the recipient not responding to the medication.

14.   Some commercial agencies do not allow negotiations. In a 2006 interview, the founder of the second major egg agency on the West Coast explained how she had recently revised her fee structure by drawing on her experience with sliding scales as a therapist.

> We wanted to be able to stay in business, but the costs were so high that we couldn't do that without raising our fees. We didn't want to raise our fees all over. We knew that donors were getting higher and higher and higher fees. It was like three or four years ago when the donor fees were going way up. A couple of people just defected: "I'm gonna get 25,000 [dollars], why should I do it for 10 [thousand dollars]?" I understood that. So if we keep this model of people who want to help, let's really hit the nail on the head with that, but let's also take certain people and spoil them. Let's tell them how wonderful they are, treat them like really nicely, give them gifts and massages and chocolates and stuff like that. We can raise the fee a certain amount, but I think we'll engender loyalty if we do these nice things for them and give them the human experience. I don't think they're all going to leave, [because] "well I can get five extra there." So that's what we did, and it helped us to keep certain clients that couldn't afford to pay. We even have a new thing called a fast track, which is an incredibly low fee for both donor and agency for people who really can't afford to do egg donation. We're working absolutely at cost, and the donor's taking a lower fee. And we did keep donors' fees down. I'm not saying they're not high, but we haven't gone past a certain fee, and I feel really proud of that, because I know a lot of places, they'll bid, or they'll say "Let the donor make her fee." We really set the donors' fees.

As of 2008, this program pays first-time donors $5,500. Donors who are considered more desirable receive $6,500 for their first cycle, and for these women, recipients are charged an extra $1,500 to pay for gifts and the marketing required to recruit "this caliber of women." All donors receive an additional $2,000 for each completed cycle.

15.   Debora Spar (2006, xvi), a professor at Harvard Business School, wrote:

> It is reasonable to assume, for example, that eggs will always cost more than sperm, because egg extraction is considerably more complicated (and potentially dangerous) than sperm donation. . . . Yet this kind of predictable variation does not explain the

range of prices that prevail in the baby market. Eggs, for example, cost far more than sperm—$4,500 versus $300 on average, and $50,000 versus $2,950 for the top end of the market. Why are parents willing to pay such high premiums for eggs? . . . Such variation cannot be explained by the customary laws of supply and demand. For the baby market does not operate like other markets do. There are differential prices that make little sense; scale economies that don't bring lower costs; and customers who will literally pay whatever they possibly can.

It is important to note that the prices Spar lists are not quite referring to the same good: $4,500 is the average fee for an egg donor to complete a cycle, which can produce anywhere from a few eggs to as many as thirty or forty, and $300 is the average cost of one vial of sperm. The sperm donor's fee is actually much less, $75 or $100 per deposit, and a single deposit can be split into as many as nine vials. Additionally, there are program fees on top of these costs for those who go through an egg agency or sperm bank.

16.   It is possible that women with posted profiles will never be chosen by recipients, just as it is possible that sperm banks may find it difficult to sell vials from particular donors. Another way to gauge supply, in sperm banks at least, would be to count the total number of vials available for purchase. However, recipients generally purchase genetic material by first choosing a donor, who may have any number of vials available, so the total number of donors is probably a more useful gauge of supply.

17.   To maintain comparability, fee information and number of donors per program are based on 2002 data, with the exception of Gametes Inc. data, which are from 2006. University Fertility Services is not included because the numbers are too small for any given year.

18.   Sperm banks do charge more for vials of "washed" sperm. This procedure is required for intrauterine insemination but is not associated with a donor's characteristics.

19.   Rapp (2000, xiv).

20.   In reading psychological evaluations of egg donors in University Fertility Services' files, I found a few in which the psychologist recommended that the applicant be rejected because she expressed more financial than altruistic motivations. In some cases, though, these women were still allowed to donate. Sperm donors were not subject to psychological screening, so there is no equivalent documentation of their motivations.

21.   Future technological changes will undoubtedly influence the market for sex cells. For example, the possibility of frozen egg banks will make the storage of eggs and sperm more parallel, but it is unlikely to change the need for women to take fertility medications and for men to masturbate. Also, it will not revolutionize gendered norms of parenting. So just as the emerging technologies of insemination and IVF were enacted in keeping with the gendered, raced, and

classed cultural norms of the time, so too will future developments in reproductive technology.

3. PRODUCING EGGS AND SPERM

1. Once the eggs are removed, an egg donor is finished, but an infertile woman must wait a few days to see if fertilization occurs in the laboratory. If it does, the embryos are implanted in her uterus, and she waits to see if pregnancy occurs.

2. Franklin (1997, 130; 106; 114).

3. Becker (2000, 55). See also Thompson (2005, Chapter 6).

4. "Aborted cycles," in which the donor had begun but ceased taking fertility medications before the egg retrieval, are calculated as 0.5.

5. On average, it had been eighteen months between a woman's *first* cycle and our interview.

6. Two donors from two different programs, Tiffany and Kim, had not yet donated. Both could accurately describe what would happen in the cycle, and each expected to experience some cramping, "like PMS." Both pointed out that they were not afraid of needles, so they did not think the shots would be a "big deal."

7. I do not use her pseudonym to protect her identity.

8. Only one woman said she was absolutely not willing to donate again; she had donated four times several years before our interview. The other women were not sure if they would be interested in donating again but all said they would consider it.

9. Laqueur (2004).

10. Laumann et al. (1994, 69).

11. Laumann et al. (1994, 81–86).

12. Michael et al. (1994, 155) reports results from Laumann et al. (1994)'s study but is intended for a general audience.

13. Inhorn (2007, 47). See also Thompson (2005, Chapter 4).

14. CryoCorp put out a sign-up sheet, but none of the donors were willing to be interviewed, and University Fertility Services no longer had active sperm donors at the time of my research.

15. *A methodological note:* In the course of doing this research, I have often been asked about what it is like to be a woman interviewing men about masturbation. I did feel some trepidation preparing for my first interview with a sperm donor, but it was not unlike the trepidation I felt before meeting with a nationally known physician or in cold-calling a donation program. My interview schedule did not include specific prompts about what happened in the donation

room, but in that first interview, Ethan responded to an open-ended question about how donation fits into his daily life by offering the extremely detailed description of producing a sample that is excerpted in this section. Thus, from that very first interview, I was convinced that the reason social scientists know so little about men's experiences of masturbation, and of reproduction more generally, is because we do not ask. I did continue to refrain from asking specific questions about masturbation, instead allowing those who wished to elaborate to do so in response to other questions. In several cases, these elaborations came at the end of the interview, when men would respond to my standard closing question, "Is there anything else you'd like to add?" by saying something along the lines of "I don't know how much detail you want, but . . ." It is also noteworthy that men from Western Sperm Bank tended to go into more detail, which could be due to the fact that those interviews were longer and conducted outside the sperm bank.

16. Several men mentioned the thin doors. One donor described overhearing the donor manager say to the laboratory technician that she was just "waiting for one more" before going to lunch, so he tried to hurry up and finish.

17. There is no significant difference between the average weekly visits of donors at Gametes Inc. and Western Sperm Bank.

18. The four youngest egg donors (all under twenty-two years of age) were the only ones to mention abstinence, and they did so briefly. Heather noted, "I told my boyfriend that I was thinking about doing [egg donation]. He was supportive. I told him you have to go for a period of abstinence. You can't even really be anywhere remotely close to each other, or I'm popping out eight kids at once [laughs]."

19. Michael et al. (1994, 155).

20. Thompson (2005, Chapter 2) summarizes the history of feminist scholarship on IVF.

21. Konrad (2005, 61–66). Emphasis added.

22. On the social construction of the body, see Turner (1984), Butler (1993), and Fausto-Sterling (2000).

23. See, for example, Scheper-Hughes and Lock (1987), Williams (1998), Wilkinson (1996), and Fausto-Sterling (2005).

4. BEING A PAID DONOR

1. Classic works include Snow et al. (1986), Swidler (1986), Swidler (2001), and Lamont (1992).

2. Healy (2006, 17). Healy provides several examples of how gift rhetoric results in particular organizational configurations, including a comparison of

how voluntary blood banks and for-profit plasma companies responded to the emerging risk of HIV in the 1980s. Healy construes this episode as a natural experiment of Titmuss' argument that relying on altruism produces safer blood and is morally preferable to for-profit systems. Blood bank staffers, who characterized blood as a gift, resisted new screening measures for fear of alienating loyal donors, thereby endangering the blood supply. Plasma companies, who perceived plasma as a commodity, had little compunction about jettisoning paid providers but responded to financial incentives to keep older (and contaminated) batches of plasma on the market. In decoupling the type of exchange from its effects, Healy successfully undermines normative assumptions about the evils of the marketplace and the benefits of gift exchange by showing the failures of both to protect the blood supply.

3. Beyond the donors interviewed for this study, additional evidence that egg and sperm donors are motivated by money comes from the psychological literature (Schover et al. 1991 and Schover, Rothmann, and Collins 1992) and the fact that there is a shortage of people willing to donate in countries where compensation is either minimal or not allowed, including Australia, Canada, and the United Kingdom (Mundy 2007, 186–7). There have also been news reports in the United States of a sharp increase in the number of applicants to egg agencies following the economic crisis of 2008 (Nichols and Moore 2009).

4. I did not ask donors about religion or spirituality, but there are linguistic hints of this being important in a few interviews, as when Ben, who is Jewish, uses the term "blessed" or when Ryan refers to the "miracle" of having a child.

5. Since women donated at different times and in different programs, the fees of individual egg donors are not directly comparable to one another.

6. It is interesting to note that Gretchen did not tell the friends to whom she had donated that she signed on with an egg agency. "Part of me thinks that Barbara and Phil would think it would lessen our bond. It is kind of a special bond. I'm going to be in their life the rest of their life, and even if they try to forget about me, every time they look at their kid, that kid would not be there, or at least partially, except for me. So, I wonder if Barbara might think I was cheapening it, if that makes sense."

7. Egg donors' reluctance to ask for higher fees reflects a broader trend of gender differences in negotiating strategies, which have been studied extensively in the context of salary negotiations (Babcock and Laschever 2003 and Stuhlmacher and Walters 1999).

8. See Zelizer (1997) on earmarking money.

9. I interviewed each donor once (with the exception of Ethan, who I interviewed a second time), so this model is not based on temporal data. However, I structured the interviews chronologically, first asking how they originally

heard about donation, what led them to contact the donation program, and about their initial meetings with staff before asking where donation fits into daily life, how they spend the money, and how gamete donation compares to blood and organ donation, paid employment, and parenthood. In this way, I can compare what originally sparked their interest in donation with how they talk about what kind of activity it is. Also, I conducted interviews with women and men at various stages in the process of donation, and there were differences in how those who were relatively new talked about it compared to those who had been donating longer, which provides additional support for the finding that donors' conceptualizations of donation shifts over time.

10.   Three men and seven women did not use the specific terms "gift" and "job," so I rely on other indicators of how they conceptualize donation. The three men were all students who cataloged sperm donation alongside their other forms of low-wage employment, suggesting that they do consider it a job. Two women's descriptions echoed those of egg donors who did call donation a gift, but five women were more outspoken about their interest in the money. Nevertheless, these five still did not call donation a job. Of the donors who were primarily interested in helping recipients, none called donation a job, and all three women in that category called donation a gift.

11.   Three-quarters of the women, compared to just 10% of the men, referenced the money that recipients are spending on donation. Half the women and 15% of the men talked about the recipients' emotional investment.

12.   About half the women and men had donated blood.

13.   Ben was originally an anonymous donor, but given that donation was a charitable project for him, he changed his status to identity-release when bank staff told him that people would be more likely to purchase his samples. He did not make this decision lightly, consulting his family and thinking it over for quite some time.

14.   It is worth noting that all three of the men quoted here (Dennis, Ben, and Ethan) donated at Western Sperm Bank, where I did longer interviews than at Gametes Inc. This may have allowed time for these issues to emerge. However, hints of similar feelings also appeared in several interviews with men at Gametes Inc.

15.   It is interesting to note that elsewhere in the interview, Nicole places limits on this sort of conceptualization, stating that she would not be a surrogate mother, because it is too much like prostitution.

16.   According to Novaes (1985, 573), French sperm banks require sperm donors to be married and have at least one child. Men do not receive any compensation, and the donation is framed as a "gift from one couple to another." This provides additional evidence for the claim that there is nothing inherent in

biology or technology that produces particular market configurations, and it would be interesting to examine the effects of this alternative framework for sperm donors' experiences of assisted reproduction.

5. DEFINING CONNECTIONS

1. Studies of recipients usually focus on heterosexual couples (Becker 2000, Becker, Butler, and Nachtigall 2005, Thompson 2005, Hargreaves 2006, and Grace and Daniels 2007), but there is a growing literature on lesbians and single women who are using reproductive technologies to have children (Haimes and Weiner 2000, Mamo 2007, and Pelka 2009). Empirical studies of offspring are still few and far between (Scheib, Riordan, and Rubin 2005 and Jadva et al. 2009).

2. Daniels and Taylor (1993).

3. Most studies of donors are based on psychological surveys (e.g., Schover et al. 1991, Schover, Rothmann, and Collins 1992, Lui et al. 1995, and Fielding et al. 1998). Daniels (1998) reviews seven studies of egg donors and ten studies of sperm donors. In one of the few qualitative studies of donors, Konrad (2005) interviews egg donors and recipients in Britain, where donors are usually married mothers who are not paid.

4. Strathern (1992), Edwards et al. (1993), Franklin and MacKinnon (2001), and Inhorn and Birenbaum-Carmeli (2008).

5. Ragoné (1994) and Teman (2010).

6. More than half the men explicitly stated that offspring *are* their children, yet just a tenth of the women said this. Nearly 60% of women explicitly stated that the offspring *are not* their children, while just 15% of men did. Another indicator of how donors think about their relationship to offspring is the use of kinship language (e.g., donors referring to themselves as parents to the offspring, referring to their parents as grandparents to the offspring, or referring to their children as siblings to the offspring); 85% of men used kinship language compared to just 42% of women. Moreover, these two indicators are generally consistent. All of the donors who considered offspring to be their children as well as donors who waffled by saying that offspring are *not really* their children, used kinship language. Most donors who said that offspring are not their children did not use kinship language. And the donors who did not specify their relationship to offspring generally did not use kinship language. I merge these two indicators to categorize all donors as conceptualizing offspring as their own children (fifteen men and five women) or not (five men and fourteen women).

In considering what else (other than gender) contributes to these differing orientations, I analyzed other possible factors, including women's and men's original interest in donation, the donation program with which they were affiliated, how long they had been donating, and where they were in the course of their lives, specifically their age and whether they had children of their own. But this sample of qualitative interviews is not large enough to reveal whether there are significant differences along these lines. For example, it may be that a donor's stage in life influences feelings of connection. The donors' median age at the time of the interview was twenty-five, and sperm donors who were both younger and older were equally likely to think of offspring as their children. Younger egg donors were a little less likely than older egg donors to consider offspring their children. However, age and parental status were correlated (and more of the egg donors were parents), and donors who had children of their own spoke in more detail about offspring. So although there are some faint patterns, it is difficult to tease them out in such a small sample. However, none of these attributes appeared so powerful as gender in predicting donors' feelings of connection (or lack thereof) to offspring.

7. See note 6 above.

8. Although one might expect family members to raise issues of relatedness, donors were just as likely to hear this sort of question from friends.

9. This is quite common among surrogates, who use similar language to egg donors in making sure that they, too, are not categorized as mothers. For example, surrogates will describe their contribution as "just a womb," and they also reference the house-painting analogy that Carla discusses earlier in this section (Teman 2010, Teman personal communication 2010).

10. I did not interview donors at the other West Coast sperm bank, CryoCorp.

11. Five egg donors reported that recipients had become pregnant (a total of one or two pregnancies per donor), four egg donors knew that recipients had given birth (a total of one or two children per donor), and one egg donor said the recipient had not become pregnant and had frozen the embryos for a future attempt. Three sperm donors were told that no pregnancies had been reported to the bank, and three said that recipients had given birth (a total of two to four children per donor). Both of the men who donated more than a decade before our interview had been asked to make additional deposits years later for recipients who wanted to conceive a full sibling for children they already had. It is important to note that most of the women and men I interviewed are still actively donating, so the number of pregnancies and offspring is likely to increase.

12. Additional evidence for this claim comes from the interviews with egg donors at Gametes Inc., who were not told what happens with their donations; they are less likely than women at other egg agencies to mention the possibility that recipients may not become pregnant.

13. In contrast to Carla's quote above, in which she references the offspring as female, Greg assumes the child will be male.

14. Gametes Inc.'s proportion refers only to those profiles posted after 2001, when the bank began offering identity release as an option.

15. Scheib and Cushing (2007).

16. To doublecheck this finding, a research assistant recoded more than 300 pages of interview text, which I had originally categorized as "gametes/recipients/offspring," solely with this question in mind. In referencing what it is that they donate to recipients, nearly 90% of women mentioned eggs, but just about half the men discussed their donation in terms of sperm. Almost half the women suggested that their donation made it possible for recipients to experience pregnancy, yet just 10% of men did. Nearly everyone conceptualized his or her donation in terms of children. But women were twice as likely to reference the probabilistic nature of their donation; about 80% of women specified that they were providing recipients a "chance" or "opportunity" to be pregnant or have children, thus demonstrating awareness that recipients may not become pregnant or that the pregnancy may not end with a birth.

17. Indeed, there are long-standing concerns about paternity disputes in sperm donation, and these are reflected in the legal battles of the mid-1900s that worried members of the nascent ASRM as well as in the lesbian-friendly Western Sperm Bank's decision to set eighteen as an age minimum for offspring to receive donors' identifying information.

18. See Daniels (2006, 11–30) for a brief overview of how women's and men's contributions to reproduction have been understood since the ancient Greeks.

19. Delaney (1986, 495). See also Franklin (1997).

20. Hayes 1996. These expectations of women are made especially clear during pregnancy, as evident in Elizabeth Armstrong's research on fetal alcohol syndrome (2003) and Laura Gomez' research on "crack babies" in the 1980s (1997).

CONCLUSION

1. See, for example, Spar (2006). Then a professor at Harvard Business School, the publication of Spar's book was covered by a wide range of media outlets, including CBS News, *The Economist,* and the *New England Journal of Medicine.* In what was deemed a provocative thesis, she contends that there is a "flourishing market for both children and their component parts. . . . [This book] does not insist that this market is either good or evil. It simply argues that it exists" (xv). Chapter by chapter, Spar investigated the structure of the "baby trade," from adoption to surrogacy and egg and sperm donation.

[E]very day, in nearly every country, infants and children are indeed being sold. . . . Understandably, most of these transactions appear to be above or beyond the market. Orphaned children, for example, are never "sold"; they're simply "matched" with "forever families." Eggs are "donated," and surrogate mothers offer their services to help the infertile. Certainly, the rhetoric that surrounds these transactions has nothing to do with markets or prices or profits. Quite possibly, the people who undertake them want only to help. *But neither the rhetoric nor the motive can change the underlying activity.* When parents buy eggs or sperm; when they contract with surrogates; when they choose a child to adopt or an embryo to implant, they are doing business. Firms are making money, customers are making choices, and children—for better or worse—are being sold (x-xi, emphasis added).

Spar does depart from the traditional view of commodification as inherently harmful, declining to take a normative position on whether the baby business is "good or evil." Nonetheless, she relies on the same dichotomous view of economic activity as separate from social life found in such classics as Richard Titmuss' book on blood donation, *The Gift Relationship.*

2. See Gal and Kligman (2000, Chapter 3) for a discussion of public/private as a fractal distinction.

3. Hays (1996, 174).

4. Collins (2000) and Roberts (1997).

5. Duster (2003).

6. Rose and Lewis (2005).

7. Other related markets include care work and domestic work, which have been the subject of much more empirical research. As noted in a recent interdisciplinary collection (Boris and Parreñas 2010), it is important to bring together scholarship on these disparate kinds of "intimate labors" to generate new thinking about the process and experience of bodily commodification.

8. Schicktanz, Schweda, and Wohlke (2010).

9. Healy (2006).

10. Scheper-Hughes (2001a).

11. Teman (2010) and Pande (2010).

12. Ragoné (1994) and Teman (2010).

13. Logan (2010).

14. Kulick (1998).

15. Bernstein (2007, 179–180). Emphasis in original.

16. Sharp (2000).

17. Reardon (2001), Wailoo and Pemberton (2006), Bolnick et al. (2007), Fullwiley (2007), Bolnick (2008), and Nelson (2008).

18. Rapp (2000).

Bibliography

Abolafia, Mitchel. 1996. *Making Markets: Opportunism and Restraint on Wall Street*. Cambridge, MA: Harvard University Press.

Acker, Joan. 1990. "Hierarchies, Jobs, Bodies: A Theory of Gendered Organizations." *Gender and Society* 4: 139–58.

Almeling, Rene. 2006. " 'Why do you want to be a donor?': Gender and the Production of Altruism in Egg and Sperm Donation." *New Genetics and Society* 25: 143–57.

———. 2007. "Selling Genes, Selling Gender: Egg Agencies, Sperm Banks, and the Medical Market in Genetic Material." *American Sociological Review* 72: 319–40.

———. 2009. "Gender and the Value of Bodily Goods: Commodification in Egg and Sperm Donation." *Law and Contemporary Problems* 72: 37–58.

American College of Obstetricians and Gynecologists. 2006. *Multiple Pregnancy and Birth: Considering Fertility Treatments*, www.acog.org.

Ansbacher, Rudi. 1978. "Artificial Insemination with Frozen Spermatozoa." *Fertility and Sterility* 29: 375–79.

Appadurai, Arjun. 1986. *The Social Life of Things: Commodities in Cultural Perspective*. Cambridge: Cambridge University Press.

Armstrong, Elizabeth. 2003. *Conceiving Risk, Bearing Responsibility: Fetal Alcohol Syndrome and the Diagnosis of Moral Disorder*. Baltimore: Johns Hopkins University Press.

Babcock, Linda and Sara Laschever. 2003. *Women Don't Ask: Negotiation and the Gender Divide*. Princeton, NJ: Princeton University Press.

Baker, Wayne. 1984. "The Social Structure of a National Securities Market." *American Journal of Sociology* 89: 775–811.

Barad, D., and B. Cohen. 1996. "Oocyte Donation Program at Montefiore Medical Center, Albert Einstein." In *New Ways of Making Babies: The Case of Egg Donation*, edited by C. B. Cohen. Bloomington: Indiana University Press.

Becker, Gary S. and Julio Jorge Elias. 2007. "Introducing Incentives in the Market for Live and Cadaveric Organ Donations." *Journal of Economic Perspectives* 21: 3–24.

Becker, Gay. 2000. *The Elusive Embryo: How Women and Men Approach New Reproductive Technologies*. Berkeley: University of California Press.

Becker, Gay, Anneliese Butler, and Robert Nachtigall. 2005. "Resemblance Talk: A Challenge for Parents Whose Children Were Conceived with Donor Gametes in the U.S." *Social Science and Medicine* 61: 1300–1309.

Beisel, Nicola and Tamara Kay. 2004. "Abortion, Race, and Gender in Nineteenth-Century America." *American Sociological Review* 69: 498–518.

Bell, Susan. 2009. *DES Daughters: Embodied Knowledge and the Transformation of Women's Health Politics*. Philadelphia: Temple University Press.

Bergh, Paul. 1999. "Indecent Proposal: $5,000 is Not 'Reasonable Compensation' for Oocyte Donors—A Reply." *Fertility and Sterility* 71: 9–10.

Bernstein, Elizabeth. 2007. *Temporarily Yours: Intimacy, Authenticity, and the Commerce of Sex*. Chicago: University of Chicago Press.

Blair-Loy, Mary. 2003. *Competing Devotions: Career and Family Among Women Executives*. Cambridge, MA: Harvard University Press.

Bolnick, Deborah. 2008. "Individual Ancestry Inference and the Reification of Race as a Biological Phenomenon." In *Revisiting Race in a Genomic Age*, edited by Barbara Koenig, Sandra Soo-Jin Lee, and Sarah Richardson. New Brunswick, NJ: Rutgers University Press.

Bolnick, D. A., D. Fullwiley, T. Duster, R. S. Cooper, J. H. Fujimura, J. Kahn, J. S. Kaufman, J. Marks, A. Morning, A. Nelson, P. Ossorio, J. Reardon, S.M. Reverby, and K. TallBear. 2007. "The Science and Business of Genetic Ancestry Testing." *Science* 318: 399–400.

Boris, Eileen and Rhacel Salazar Parreñas. 2010. *Intimate Labors: Cultures, Technologies, and the Politics of Care*. Stanford, CA: Stanford University Press.

Boston Women's Health Book Collective. 2008 [1971]. *Our Bodies, Ourselves*. New York: Simon and Schuster.

Braverman, Andrea. 1993. "Survey Results on the Current Practice of Ovum Donation." *Fertility and Sterility* 59: 1216–20.

Braverman, Andrea and Stephen Corson. 1995. "Factors Related to Preferences in Gamete Donor Sources." *Fertility and Sterility* 63: 543–59.

Browner, Carole and Nancy Press. 1995. "The Normalization of Prenatal Diagnostic Screening." In *Conceiving the New World Order: The Global Politics of Reproduction*, edited by F. Ginsburg and R. Rapp. Berkeley: University of California Press.

Butler, Judith. 1993. *Bodies that Matter: On the Discursive Limits of Sex*. New York: Routledge.

Carrier, James. 1995. *Gifts and Commodities: Exchange and Western Capitalism since 1700*. New York: Routledge.

Centers for Disease Control and Prevention, American Society for Reproductive Medicine, and Society for Assisted Reproductive Technology. 2008. *2006 Assisted Reproductive Technology Success Rates: National Summary and Fertility Clinic Reports*. Atlanta: U.S. Department of Health and Human Services, Centers for Disease Control and Prevention.

Chodorow, Nancy. 1978. *The Reproduction of Mothering: Psychoanalysis and the Sociology of Gender*. Berkeley: University of California Press.

Clarke, Adele. 1998. *Disciplining Reproduction: Modernity, American Life Sciences, and "The Problems of Sex."* Berkeley: University of California Press.

Collins, Patricia Hill. 2000 [1990]. *Black Feminist Thought: Knowledge, Consciousness, and the Politics of Empowerment*. New York: Routledge.

Coltrane, Scott. 1996. *Family Man: Fatherhood, Housework, and Gender Equity*. New York: Oxford University Press.

Connell, Robert. 1987. *Gender and Power*. Stanford, CA: Stanford University Press.

Conrad, Peter. 2007. *The Medicalization of Society: On the Transformation of Human Conditions into Treatable Disorders*. Baltimore: Johns Hopkins University Press.

Conrad, Peter and Valerie Leiter. 2004. "Medicalization, Markets, and Consumers." *Journal of Health and Social Behavior* 45: 158–76.

Covington, Sharon and William Gibbons. 2007. "What is Happening to the Price of Eggs?" *Fertility and Sterility* 87: 1001–1004.

Daniels, Cynthia. 2006. *Exposing Men: The Science and Politics of Male Reproduction*. New York: Oxford University Press.

Daniels, Ken. 1998. "The Semen Providers." In *Donor Insemination: International Social Science Perspectives*, edited by K. Daniels and E. Haimes. Cambridge: Cambridge University Press.

Daniels, Ken and Erica Haimes, eds. 1998. *Donor Insemination: International Social Science Perspectives*. Cambridge: Cambridge University Press.

Daniels, Ken and Karyn Taylor. 1993. "Secrecy and Openness in Donor Insemination." *Politics and the Life Sciences* 12: 155–70.

Davis, M. Edward. 1956. "Statement of the American Society for the Study of Sterility Approving Donor Insemination." *Fertility and Sterility* 7: 101–102.

De Beauvoir, Simone. 1989 [1952]. *The Second Sex*. New York: Vintage.

Delaney, Carol. 1986. "The Meaning of Paternity and the Virgin Birth Debate." *Man* 21: 494–513.

Duka, Walter and Alan DeCherney. 1994. *From the Beginning: A History of the American Fertility Society 1944–1994*. Birmingham, AL: American Fertility Society.

Duster, Troy. 2003 [1990]. *Backdoor to Eugenics*. New York: Routledge.

Eastlund, D. Ted and David Stroncek. 1993. "Letter to the Editor: More on Compensating Egg Donors." *New England Journal of Medicine* 329: 278.

Edwards, Jeanette, Sarah Franklin, Eric Hirsch, Frances Price, and Marilyn Strathern. 1993. *Technologies of Procreation: Kinship in the Age of Assisted Conception*. Manchester: Manchester University Press.

Elton, Catherine. March 31, 2009. "As Egg Donations Mount, So Do Health Concerns." *Time Magazine*.

England, Paula and Nancy Folbre. 2005. "Gender and Economic Sociology." In *The Handbook of Economic Sociology*, edited by N. Smelser and R. Swedberg. Princeton, NJ: Princeton University Press.

Espeland, Wendy. 1984. "Blood and Money: Exploiting the Embodied Self." In *The Existential Self in Society*, edited by J. Kotarba and A. Fontana. Chicago: University of Chicago Press.

Ethics Committee of the American Society for Reproductive Medicine. 2000. "Financial Incentives in Recruitment of Oocyte Donors." *Fertility and Sterility* 74: 216–20.

Fausto-Sterling, Anne. 2000. *Sexing the Body: Gender Politics and the Construction of the Body*. New York: Basic Books.

———. 2005. "The Bare Bones of Sex: Part 1—Sex and Gender." *Signs: Journal of Women in Culture and Society* 30: 1491–1527.

Fielding, Dorothy, Sarah Handley, Lindsay Duqueno, Sue Weaver, and Steve Lui. 1998. "Motivation Attitudes and Experience of Donation: A Follow-Up of Women Donating Eggs in Assisted Conception Treatment." *Journal of Community and Applied Social Psychology* 8: 245–48.

Foster-Fraser, Kathryn Leslie. 1990. "Male Donors' Personality Characteristics, Parental Relationships, and Motivations to Participate in Artificial Insemination." PhD diss., California School of Professional Psychology, Berkeley/Alameda, Proquest Dissertations and Theses, AAT 9020079.

Franklin, Sarah. 1997. *Embodied Progress: A Cultural Account of Assisted Conception*. London: Routledge.

Franklin, Sarah and Susan McKinnon. 2001. *Relative Values: Reconfiguring Kinship Studies*. Durham, NC: Duke University Press.

Freidson, Eliot. 1970. *Profession of Medicine: A Study of the Sociology of Applied Knowledge*. New York: Harper and Row.

Friese, Carrie. 2009. "Models of Cloning, Models for the Zoo: Rethinking the Sociological Significance of Cloned Animals." *BioSocieties* 4: 367–90.

Fullwiley, Duana. 2007. "The Molecularization of Race: Institutionalizing Racial Difference in Pharmacogenetics Practice." *Science as Culture* 16: 1–30.

Gal, Susan and Gail Kligman. 2000. *The Politics of Gender after Socialism: A Comparative-Historical Essay*. Princeton, NJ: Princeton University Press.

German, E.K., T. Mukherjee, D. Osborne, and A.B. Copperman. 2001. "Does Increasing Ovum Donor Compensation Lead to Differences in Donor Characteristics?" *Fertility and Sterility* 76: 75–79.

Ginsburg, Faye and Rayna Rapp. 1995. *Conceiving the New World Order: The Global Politics of Reproduction*. Berkeley: University of California Press.

Gomez, Laura. 1997. *Misconceiving Mothers: Legislators, Prosecutors, and the Politics of Prenatal Drug Exposure*. Philadelphia: Temple University Press.

Gordon, Linda. 1976. *Woman's Body, Woman's Right: A Social History of Birth Control in America*. New York: Viking Press.

Gorrill, Marsha, Lisa Johnson, Phillip Patton, and Kenneth Burry. 2001. "Oocyte Donor Screening: The Selection Process and Cost Analysis." *Fertility and Sterility* 75: 400–404.

Grace, Victoria M. and Ken R. Daniels. 2007. "The (Ir)relevance of Genetics: Engendering Parallel Worlds of Procreation and Reproduction." *Sociology of Health and Illness* 29: 692–710.

Gregory, C.A. 1982. *Gifts and Commodities*. London: Academic Press.

Guttmacher, Alan. 1958. "Artificial Insemination: Genetic, Legal, and Ethical Implications: A Symposium." *Fertility and Sterility* 9: 368–75.

Guttmacher, Alan, John Haman, and John MacLeod. 1950. "The Use of Donors for Artificial Insemination: A Survey of Current Practices." *Fertility and Sterility* 1: 264–70.

Haimes, Erica. 1993. "Issues of Gender in Gamete Donation." *Social Science and Medicine* 3: 85–93.

Haimes, Erica and Kate Weiner. 2000. " 'Everybody's got a dad . . .' Issues for Lesbian Families in the Management of Donor Insemination." *Sociology of Health and Illness* 22: 477–99.

Hard, Addison. 1909. "Artificial Impregnation." *The Medical World* April: 163–64.

Hargreaves, Katrina. 2006. "Constructing Families and Kinship through Donor Insemination." *Sociology of Health and Illness* 28: 261–83.

Hays, Sharon. 1996. *The Cultural Contradictions of Motherhood*. New Haven, CT and London: Yale University Press.

Healy, Kieran. 2006. *Last Best Gifts: Altruism and the Market for Human Blood and Organs*. Chicago: University of Chicago Press.

Hochschild, Arlie. 1983. *The Managed Heart: Commercialization of Human Feeling*. Berkeley: University of California Press.

Hopkins, Jim. March 16, 2006. "Egg-Donor Business Booms on Campuses." *USA Today*, 1A.

Hondagneu-Sotelo, Pierrette. 2001. *Domestica: Immigrant Workers Cleaning and Caring in the Shadow of Affluence*. Berkeley: University of California Press.

Inhorn, Marcia. 2007. "Masturbation, Semen Collection, and Men's IVF Experiences: Anxieties in the Muslim World." *Body and Society* 13: 37–53.

Inhorn, Marcia and Daphna Birenbaum-Carmeli. 2008. "Assisted Reproductive Technologies and Culture Change." *Annual Review of Anthropology* 37: 177–96.

Jadva, Vasanti, Tabitha Freeman, Wendy Kramer, and Susan Golombok. 2009. "The Experiences of Adolescents and Adults Conceived by Sperm Donation: Comparisons by Age of Disclosure and Family Type." *Human Reproduction* 24: 1909–19.

Jordan, Brigitte. 1983. *Birth in Four Cultures*. Montreal: Eden Press.

Kanter, Rosabeth M. 1977. *Men and Women of the Corporation*. New York: Basic Books.

Katz Rothman, Barbara. 1986. *The Tentative Pregnancy: Prenatal Diagnosis and the Future of Motherhood*. New York: Viking.

Kennard, Elizabeth, Robert Collins, Josef Blankstein, Leslie Schover, George Kanoti, Joann Reiss, and Martin Quigley. 1989. "A Program for Matched, Anonymous Oocyte Donation." *Fertility and Sterility* 51: 655–60.

Kimmel, Michael. 2006. *Manhood in America: A Cultural History*. New York: Oxford University Press.

Kligman, Gail. 1998. *The Politics of Duplicity: Controlling Reproduction in Ceausescu's Romania*. Berkeley: University of California Press.

Kolata, Gina. February 25, 1998. "Price of Donor Eggs Soars, Setting off a Debate on Ethics." *New York Times*.

Konrad, Monica. 2005. *Nameless Relations: Anonymity, Melanesia, and Reproductive Gift Exchange between British Ova Donors and Recipients*. New York: Berghahn Books.

Kulick, Don. 1998. *Travesti: Sex, Gender, and Culture among Brazilian Transgendered Prostitutes*. Chicago: University of Chicago Press.

Lamont, Michèle. 1992. *Money, Morals, and Manners: The Culture of the French and American Upper-Middle Class*. Chicago: University of Chicago Press.

Landes, Elisabeth M. and Richard A. Posner. 1978. "The Economics of the Baby Shortage." *The Journal of Legal Studies* 7: 323–48.

Laqueur, Thomas W. 2004. *Solitary Sex: A Cultural History of Masturbation*. New York: Zone Books.

Laumann, Edward, John Gagnon, Robert Michael, and Stuart Michaels. 1994. *The Social Organization of Sexuality: Sexual Practices in the United States*. Chicago: University of Chicago Press.

Lessor, Roberta, Nancyann Cervantes, Nadine O'Connor, Jose Balmaceda, and Ricardo Asch. 1993. "An Analysis of Social and Psychological Characteristics of Women Volunteering To Become Oocyte Donors." *Fertility and Sterility* 59: 65–71.

Light, Donald. 1993. "Countervailing Powers: The Changing Character of the Medical Profession in the United States." In *The Changing Character of the Medical Profession*, edited by F. Hafferty and J. McKinley. New York: Oxford University Press.

———. 2004. "Ironies of Successes: A New History of the American Health Care System." *Journal of Health and Social Behavior* 45: 1–24.

Logan, Trevon D. 2010. "Personal Characteristics, Sexual Behaviors, and Male Sex Work: A Quantitative Approach." *American Sociological Review* 75: 679–704.

Lopez, Steven. 2006. "Emotional Labor and Organized Emotional Care: Conceptualizing Nursing Home Care Work." *Work and Occupations* 33: 133–60.

Lui, S. C., S.M. Weaver, J. Robinson, M. Debono, M. Nieland, S.R. Killick, and D.M. Hay. 1995. "Survey of Semen Donor Attitudes." *Human Reproduction* 10: 234–38.

Luker, Kristen. 1984. *Abortion and the Politics of Motherhood*. Berkeley: University of California Press.

Lutgen, Peter, Alan Trounson, John Leeton, Jock Findlay, Carl Wood, and Peter Renou. 1984. "The Establishment and Maintenance of a Pregnancy Using *In vitro* Fertilization and Embryo Donation in a Patient with Primary Ovarian Failure." *Nature* 307: 174–75.

Mamo, Laura. 2007. *Queering Reproduction: Achieving Pregnancy in the Age of Technoscience*. Durham, NC: Duke University Press.

Markens, Susan. 2007. *Surrogate Motherhood and the Politics of Reproduction*. Berkeley: University of California Press.

Martin, Emily. 1991. "The Egg and the Sperm: How Science Has Constructed a Romance Based on Stereotypical Male-Female Roles." *Signs: Journal of Women in Culture and Society* 16: 485–501.

Maxwell, Kara, Ina Cholst, and Zev Rosenwaks. 2008. "The Incidence of Both Serious and Minor Complications in Young Women Undergoing Oocyte Donation." *Fertility and Sterility* 90: 2165–71.

Marx, Karl. 1936. *Capital: A Critique of Political Economy*. New York: The Modern Library.

Mauss, Marcel. 1967 [1925]. *The Gift: Forms and Functions of Exchange*. New York: W.W. Norton and Co., Inc.

McKinley, John and John Stoekle. 1988. "Corporatization and the Social Transformation of Doctoring." *International Journal of Health Services* 18: 191–205.

Michael, Robert, John Gagnon, Edward Laumann, and Gina Kolata. 1994. *Sex in America: A Definitive Survey*. Boston: Warner Books, Inc.

Moore, Lisa Jean. 2007. *Sperm Counts: Overcome By Man's Most Precious Fluid*. New York: New York University Press.

Mundy, Lisa. 2007. *Everything Conceivable: How Assisted Reproduction Is Changing Men, Women, and the World*. New York: Knopf.

Murphy, Douglas. 1964. "Donor Insemination: A Study of 511 Prospective Donors." *Fertility and Sterility* 15: 528–33.

Murray, Thomas. 1996. "New Reproductive Technologies and the Family." In *New Ways of Making Babies: The Case of Egg Donation*, edited by C. Cohen. Bloomington: Indiana University Press.

Nelson, Alondra. 2008. "Bio Science: Genetic Genealogy Testing and the Pursuit of African Ancestry." *Social Studies of Science* 38: 759–78.

Nelson, Julie and Paula England. 2002. "Feminist Philosophies of Love and Work." *Hypatia* 17: 1–18.

Nichols, Michelle and Angela Moore. February 27, 2009. "In Hard Times, More U.S. Women Try to Sell Their Eggs." *Reuters Newswire*, http://www.reuters.com/article/2009/02/27/us-financial-fertility-idUSTRE51Q3LB20090227.

Novaes, Simone B. 1985. "Social Integration of Technical Innovation: Sperm Banking and AID in France and in the United States." *Social Science Information* 24: 569–84.

Nussbaum, Martha C. 1998. "'Whether from reason or prejudice': Taking Money for Bodily Services." *Journal of Legal Studies* 27: 693–724.

Ortner, Sherry. 1974. "Is Female to Male as Nature Is to Culture?" In *Woman, Culture, and Society*, edited by M. Z. Rosaldo and L. Lamphere. Stanford, CA: Stanford University Press.

Otis, Eileen M. 2008. "Beyond the Industrial Paradigm: Market-embedded Labor and the Gender Organization of Global Service Work in China." *American Sociological Review* 73: 15–36.

Pande, Amrita. 2010. "Commercial Surrogacy in India: Manufacturing a Perfect Mother-Worker." *Signs: Journal of Women in Culture and Society* 35: 969–92.

Parsons, Talcott. 1951. *The Social System*. Glencoe, IL: Free Press.

Pelka, Suzanne. 2009. "Sharing Motherhood: Maternal Jealousy among Lesbian Co-Mothers." *Journal of Homosexuality* 56: 195–217.

Peterson, Edwin. 1986. "Artificial Insemination by Donor—A New Look." *Fertility and Sterility* 46: 567–70.

Pfeffer, Naomi. 1993. *The Stork and the Syringe: A Political History of Reproductive Medicine.* Cambridge: Polity Press.

Pierce, Jennifer. 1995. *Gender Trials: Emotional Trials in Contemporary Law Firms.* Berkeley: University of California Press.

Pollitt, Katha. May 23, 1987. "The Strange Case of Baby M." *The Nation.*

Practice Committee of the American Society for Reproductive Medicine. 2008a. "Ovarian Tissue and Oocyte Preservation." *Fertility and Sterility* 90: S241–46.

Practice Committee of the American Society for Reproductive Medicine. 2008b. "Repetitive Oocyte Donation." *Fertility and Sterility* 90: S194–95.

Rabin, Roni Caryn. May 15, 2007. "As Demand for Donor Eggs Soars, High Prices Stir Ethical Concerns." *New York Times*, F6.

Radin, Margaret. 1996. *Contested Commodities: The Trouble with Trade in Sex, Children, Body Parts, and Other Things.* Cambridge, MA: Harvard University Press.

Ragoné, Heléna. 1994. *Surrogate Motherhood: Conception in the Heart.* Boulder, CO: Westview Press.

———. 1998. "Incontestable Motivations." In *Reproducing Reproduction: Kinship, Power, and Technological Innovation*, edited by S. Franklin and H. Ragoné. Philadelphia: University of Pennsylvania Press.

Rapp, Rayna. 2000. "Foreward." In *Ideologies and Technologies of Motherhood*, edited by H. Ragoné and F. W. Twine. New York: Routledge.

Reardon, Jenny. 2001. "The Human Genome Diversity Project: A Case Study in Co-Production." *Social Studies of Science* 31: 357–88.

Relman, Arnold. 1980. "The New Medical-Industrial Complex." *New England Journal of Medicine* 303: 964–70.

Richardson, Ruth. 1987. *Death, Dissection, and the Destitute.* London: Routledge & Kegan Paul.

Rindfuss, Ronald R., S. Philip Morgan, and Kate Offut. 1996. "Education and the Changing Age Pattern of American Fertility: 1963–1989." *Demography* 33: 277–90.

Roberts, Dorothy. 1997. *Killing the Black Body: Race, Reproduction, and the Meaning of Liberty.* New York: Pantheon.

Rose, Susan and Tené Lewis. 2005. "Psychosocial Factors and Cardiovascular Diseases." *Annual Review of Public Health* 26: 469–500.

Rosenwaks, Zev. 1987. "Donor Eggs: Their Application in Modern Reproductive Technologies." *Fertility and Sterility* 47: 895–909.

Rubin, Gayle. 1975. "The Traffic in Women." In *Toward an Anthropology of Women*, edited by R. Reiter. New York: Monthly Review Press.

Sauer, Mark. 1999. "Indecent Proposal: $5,000 is Not 'Reasonable Compensation' for Oocyte Donors." *Fertility and Sterility* 71: 7–8.

———. 2001. "Defining the Incidence of Serious Complications Experienced by Oocyte Donors: A Review of 1,000 Cases." *American Journal of Obstetrics and Gynecology* 184: 277–78.

Sauer, Mark and Richard Paulson. 1992. "Understanding the Current Status of Oocyte Donation in the United States: What's Really Going on Out There?" *Fertility and Sterility* 58: 16–18.

———. 1994. "Mishaps and Misfortunes: Complications that Occur in Oocyte Donation." *Fertility and Sterility* 61: 963–95.

Sauer, Mark, Richard Paulson, Thelma Macaso, Mary Francis-Hernandez, and Rogerio Lobo. 1989. "Establishment of a Nonanonymous Donor Oocyte Program: Preliminary Experience at the University of Southern California." *Fertility and Sterility* 52: 433–36.

Scheib, J.E. and R.A. Cushing. 2007. "Open-identity Donor Insemination in the United States: Is It on the Rise?" *Fertility and Sterility* 88: 231–32.

Scheib, J.E., M. Riordan, and S. Rubin. 2005. "Adolescents with Open-Identity Sperm Donors: Reports from 12–17-Year-Olds." *Human Reproduction* 20: 239–52.

Scheper-Hughes, Nancy. 2001a. "Commodity Fetishism in Organs Trafficking." *Body and Society* 7: 31–62.

———. 2001b. "Introduction: Bodies for Sale: Whole or in Parts and Commodity Fetishism in Organs Trafficking." *Body and Society* 7: 1–8.

Scheper-Hughes, Nancy and Margaret Lock. 1987. "The Mindful Body: A Prolegomenon to Future Work in Medical Anthropology." *Medical Anthropology Quarterly* 1: 6–41.

Schicktanz, Silke, Mark Schweda, and Sabine Wohlke. 2010. "Gender Issues in Living Organ Donation: Medical, Social, and Legal Aspects." In *Sex and Gender in Biomedicine: Theories, Methodologies, Results*, edited by I. Klinge and C. Wiesemann. Universitätsverlag Göttingen.

Schmidt, Matthew and Lisa Jean Moore. 1998. "Constructing a 'Good Catch,' Picking a Winner: The Development of Technosemen and the Deconstruction of the Monolithic Male." In *Cyborg Babies: From Techno-Sex to Techno-Tots*, edited by R. Davis-Floyd and J. Dumit. New York: Routledge.

Schneider, Jennifer. 2008. "Fatal Colon Cancer in a Young Egg Donor: A Physician Mother's Call for Follow-up and Research on the Long-Term Risks of Ovarian Stimulation." *Fertility and Sterility* 90: 2061.e1–e5.

Schover, Leslie, Robert Collins, Martin Quigley, Josef Blankstein, and George Kanoti. 1991. "Psychological Follow-up of Women Evaluated as Oocyte Donors." *Human Reproduction* 6: 1487–91.

Schover, L. R., S. A. Rothmann, and R. L. Collins. 1992. "The Personality and Motivation of Semen Donors: A Comparison with Oocyte Donors." *Human Reproduction* 7: 575–79.

Seibel, Machelle and Ann Kiessling. 1993. "Letter to the Editor: Compensating Egg Donors: Equal Pay for Equal Time?" *New England Journal of Medicine* 328: 737.

Sharp, Lesley. 2000. "The Commodification of the Body and its Parts." *Annual Review of Anthropology* 29: 287–328.

Sherman, J.K. 1964. "Research on Frozen Human Semen." *Fertility and Sterility* 15: 485–99.

Sherman, Rachel. 2007. *Class Acts: Service and Inequality in Luxury Hotels.* Berkeley: University of California Press.

Snow, David, E. Burke Rochford, Jr., Steven Worden, and Robert Benford. 1986. "Frame Alignment Processes, Micromobilization, and Movement Participation." *American Sociological Review* 51: 464–81.

Spar, Debora L. 2006. *The Baby Business: How Money, Science, and Politics Drive the Commerce of Conception.* Boston: Harvard Business School Press.

Starr, Paul. 1982. *The Social Transformation of American Medicine.* New York: Basic Books.

Stephen, Elizabeth Hervey and Anjani Chandra. 2006. "Declining Estimates of Infertility in the United States: 1982–2002." *Fertility and Sterility* 86: 516–23.

Strathern, Marilyn. 1992. *Reproducing the Future: Anthropology, Kinship, and the New Reproductive Technologies.* New York: Routledge.

Stuhlmacher, Alice and Amy Walters. 1999. "Gender Differences in Negotiation Outcome: A Meta-Analysis." *Personnel Psychology* 52: 653–77.

Swidler, Ann. 1986. "Culture in Action: Symbols and Strategies." *American Sociological Review* 51: 273–86.

———. 2001. *Talk of Love: How Culture Matters.* Chicago: University of Chicago Press.

Talley, Heather. 2008. *Face Work: Cultural, Technical, and Surgical Interventions for Facial "Disfigurement."* PhD diss., Sociology Department, Vanderbilt University, Nashville.

Teman, Elly. 2010. *Birthing a Mother: The Surrogate Body and the Pregnant Self.* Berkeley: University of California Press.

Thompson, Charis. 2005. *Making Parents: The Ontological Choreography of Reproductive Technologies.* Cambridge, MA: The MIT Press.

———. 2007. "Why We Should, in Fact, Pay for Egg Donation." *Regenerative Medicine* 2: 203–209.

Timmermans, Stefan. 2006. *Postmortem: How Medical Examiners Explain Suspicious Deaths.* Chicago: University of Chicago Press.

Timmermans, Stefan and Rene Almeling. 2009. "Objectification, Standardiza-
tion, and Commodification in Healthcare: A Conceptual Readjustment."
Social Science and Medicine 69: 21–27.

Titmuss, Richard. 1971. *The Gift Relationship: From Human Blood to Social Policy.*
New York: Pantheon Books.

Tompkins, Pendleton. 1950. "A New Journal." *Fertility and Sterility* 1: 1–2.

Turner, Bryan. 1984. *The Body and Society.* New York: Basil Blackwell.

United States Office of Technology Assessment (U.S. Congress). 1988. *Artificial
Insemination: Practice in the United States: Summary of a 1987 Survey—
Background Paper, OTA-13P-BA-48.* Washington, DC: U.S. Government
Printing Office.

Velthuis, Olaf. 2005. *Talking Prices: Symbolic Meanings of Prices on the Market for
Contemporary Art.* Princeton, NJ: Princeton University Press.

Waldby, Catherine and Robert Mitchell. 2006. *Tissue Economies: Blood, Organs,
and Cell Lines in Late Capitalism.* Durham, NC: Duke University Press.

Wailoo, Keith and Stephen Pemberton. 2006. *The Troubled Dream of Genetic
Medicine: Ethnicity and Innovation in Tay-Sachs, Cystic Fibrosis, and Sickle Cell
Disease.* Baltimore: Johns Hopkins University Press.

Wilkinson, Richard. 1996. *Unhealthy Societies: The Afflictions of Inequality.*
London: Routledge.

Williams, Christine. 1995. *Still a Man's World: Men Who Do Women's Work.*
Berkeley: University of California Press.

Williams, Simon. 1998. " 'Capitalizing' on Emotions? Rethinking the Inequalities in Health Debate." *Sociology* 32: 121–139.

Yanagisako, Sylvia and Jane Collier. 1990. "The Mode of Reproduction in
Anthropology." In *Theoretical Perspectives on Sexual Difference*, edited by
D. Rhode. New Haven, CT: Yale University Press.

Zelizer, Viviana. 1979. *Morals and Markets: The Development of Life Insurance in
the United States.* New York: Columbia University Press.

———. 1985. *Pricing the Priceless Child: The Changing Social Value of Children.*
New York: Basic Books.

———. 1988. "Beyond the Polemics of the Market." *Sociological Forum* 3: 614–34.

———. 1997. *The Social Meaning of Money: Pin Money, Paychecks, Poor Relief, and
Other Currencies.* Princeton, NJ: Princeton University Press.

———. 2005. *The Purchase of Intimacy.* Princeton, NJ: Princeton University Press.

Index

Text: 10/14 Palatino
Display: Univers Condensed Light 47 and Bauer Bodoni
Compositor: Westchester Book Group
Indexer: Judy Kip
Printer and binder: Maple-Vail Book Manufacturing Group

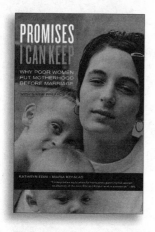

Promises I Can Keep
Why Poor Women Put Motherhood Before Marriage
KATHRYN EDIN and MARIA KEFALAS

"The most important study ever written on motherhood and marriage among low-income urban women." —**William Julius Wilson, author of** *The Bridge over the Racial Divide*

William J. Goode Best Book-Length Contribution to Family Sociology Award, American Sociological Association

$24.95 paper 978-0-520-27146-3

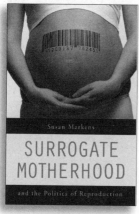

Surrogate Motherhood and the Politics of Reproduction
SUSAN MARKENS

"A fascinating history…. A timely commentary."
—*New England Journal of Medicine*

"An original, insightful book…she offers a fresh look at a vexing and timely social issue…. Feminist political sociology at its finest."
—**Monica J. Casper, author of** *The Making of the Unborn Patient*

$25.95 paper   978-0-520-25204-2

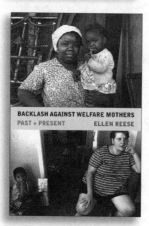

Backlash against Welfare Mothers
Past and Present
ELLEN REESE

"Carefully researched…. She documents the horrible consequences for the impoverished children and working mothers who have nothing to say about the shape of welfare…. Essential reading for everyone interested in gender, poverty, and welfare."
—*American Journal of Sociology*

$24.95 paper   978-0-520-24462-7

www.ucpress.edu